NAVIGATING MENOPAUSE

Your Essential Guide to a Life in Full Bloom

Pharm. Fatima I.Abdulkadir

Published in Nigeria by:fatiabch@gmail.com

This book stands as a tribute to the collaborative spirit of learning, growth, and shared experiences, dedicated to all women embracing menopause with grace, confidence, and vitality.

To the extraordinary women in my life—my mothers, sisters, daughters, daughters-in-law, and granddaughters—you are the heartbeats of my existence, the stars in my night sky, and the inspiration behind every word in this book. Through the tapestry of your lives, I've witnessed the strength, resilience, and boundless beauty of women in all their glory.

With love, admiration, and gratitude, this book is dedicated to you, the incredible women who light up my world. May it serve as a beacon of empowerment, a source of wisdom, and a reminder that you are all capable of achieving a life in full bloom.

With all my love,
Fatima I. Abdulkadir

CONTENTS

Disclaimer

The information provided in "Navigating Menopause: Your Essential Guide to a Life in Full Bloom" is intended for general informational purposes only. While every effort has been made to ensure the accuracy and reliability of the content, it is not to be considered a substitute for professional medical advice, diagnosis, or treatment.

Readers are encouraged to consult with qualified healthcare professionals, such as physicians, pharmacists, or other specialists, to address individual health concerns and seek personalized guidance. The author, publisher, and all related parties are not responsible for any damage or harm that may arise based on indiscriminate or discretionary use of the information provided in this book.

Additionally, the experiences and stories shared in this book are for illustrative and inspirational purposes and may not necessarily represent typical or expected outcomes.

The author and publisher disclaim any liability or responsibility for any loss or damage incurred by individuals as a result of using or relying solely on the information provided in this book. Readers should exercise their caution, discretion and judgment when applying the knowledge and recommendations from this publication to their own circumstances.By reading *"Navigating Menopause: Your Essential Guide to a Life in Full Bloom"*, readers accept and acknowledge the terms of this disclaimer.

ACKNOWLEDGMENTS

Writing a book is often a solitary endeavor; however, the support and inspiration I have received along the way have been remarkable. I want to begin by expressing my deepest gratitude to God

Almighty; for it is through His divine guidance and inspiration that this book has come to life.

First and foremost, I want to acknowledge my esteemed colleague, Pharm. Mosunmola Dosunmu. Her enlightening online seminar sparked off the inspiration for this book. Her knowledge and dedication to women's health have been a guiding light on this path; and I am profoundly grateful for her mentorship.

I also extend my heartfelt thanks to the remarkable women who generously shared their stories with me. Your openness, resilience, and experiences have enriched the content of this book and will undoubtedly resonate with countless readers. Your voices matter, and they have found a place of honor within these pages.

To my family and friends who offered unwavering encouragement and support throughout this writing process, I am deeply thankful. Your belief in me and this project has been a constant source of motivation.

Last but not least, I want to express my appreciation to the readers of this book. It is your curiosity, your thirst for knowledge, and your journey through these pages that give purpose to the words on them.

With heartfelt gratitude.

Pharm.   Fatima   I.   Abdulkadir

INTRODUCTION

The Significance of Menopause

In this book, we embark on a journey to explore the profound significance of menopause; a natural life transition that all women will encounter at some point. Understanding its importance and the need to write about it is critical to enhancing the well-being of women worldwide.

Menopause: A Universal Experience

Menopause is universal. It transcends geographic or racial barriers, cultural backgrounds or idiosyncrasies, and socioeconomic statuses. Every woman, in the course of her ascent on the biological ladder, will eventually experience menopause. This universality underscores the importance of addressing the topic comprehensively.

Health and Well-being of Women

The physical, physiological, and emotional changes that accompany menopause have a profound impact on a woman's health and overall well-being. The significance of this transition lies in the challenges it presents to women, from hormonal imbalances to an array of symptoms that can disrupt daily life. Writing about menopause is paramount to providing information and resources that empower women to navigate this phase with grace and confidence.

Empowerment through Knowledge

Knowledge is power, and it is no exception with menopause. Understanding the intricacies of menopause equips women to make informed decisions about their health and treatment options. Writing about it serves as a crucial educational tool, allowing women to actively participate in discussions with healthcare providers and tailor their choices to their specific needs and preferences.

Emotional Well-being

Menopause can be emotionally demanding, with mood swings and shifts in mental well-being. The significance of addressing these emotional challenges cannot be understated. By providing guidance and support, women can learn to navigate these emotional fluctuations effectively, maintaining good mental health and a sense of well-being.

Physical Health and Quality of Life

Menopause brings various health considerations, including bone density loss and increased susceptibility to heart disease. Understanding these health risks and adopting preventative measures is essential for maintaining physical health. Moreover, the symptoms can affect a woman's quality of life, impacting relationships, sleep, and sexual well-being. Writing about menopause offers practical insights and solutions to enhance the overall quality of life during this transition.

Reducing Misconceptions and Stigma

Misconceptions and stigmas associated with menopause can create unnecessary fear and anxiety. Addressing these myths is of great significance. Through accurate, science-based information, writing about menopause plays a vital role in dispelling these misconceptions and reducing the stigma surrounding this natural phase of life.

Empathy and Solidarity

The menopausal experience can be isolating and lonely for some women. Acknowledging the emotional and physical challenges of this transition fosters empathy and solidarity among women. It reminds them that they are not alone in their journey, encouraging the formation of supportive networks and a sense of understanding.

Career and Workplace Considerations

Menopause can significantly affect a woman's professional life; from disruptions caused by symptoms to the emotional toll it can take. Addressing these considerations is vital to helping women maintain their careers and thrive during menopause.

Positive Aging

Embracing menopause as part of the aging process is a significant aspect of this life transition. By discussing the importance of aging positively and with grace, writing about menopause can help women experience this phase of life with fulfillment and satisfaction, fostering a healthier and more positive approach to aging.

The significance of menopause is multi-faceted, encompassing women's physical and emotional well-being, empowerment through knowledge, the reduction of stigma and misconceptions, and the fostering of empathy and solidarity. Writing about menopause is of paramount importance, contributing to a more informed and supportive society for women experiencing this natural transition and encouraging a healthier and more positive approach to aging.

An Unexpected Journey: My Personal Encounter with Menopause

In my journey as a pharmacist, I've had the privilege of helping countless women navigate the challenges of menopause. I have provided advice, prescribed medications and offered support to many on their path through this profound life transition. However, what truly deepened my understanding and empathy was when I found myself facing the same journey.

I was in my early 50s when I started experiencing the telltale signs of menopause. Hot flashes became my unwanted companion, often striking at the most inconvenient times. My mood sometimes swung like a pendulum, causing me to question my emotional stability. I found myself searching for the same guidance and support that I had offered to others for years.

It was a humbling experience as the knowledge and expertise I had accumulated as a pharmacist could not shield me from the realities of menopause. The emotional ups and downs, the nights disrupted by night sweats, and the frustration of trying to manage my symptoms while maintaining a busy professional life became my new reality. I realized that menopause was more than just a clinical concept; it was a personal journey, which tested my resilience and adaptability.

This experience allowed me to connect on a deeper level with the women I had been assisting over the years. I understood firsthand the physical and emotional toll of menopause. I empathized with the challenges they faced, from making decisions about hormone therapy to managing daily life while dealing with symptoms.

My journey through menopause reinforced the importance of providing comprehensive support, education, and resources to women during this life transition. It underscored the significance of empathy and solidarity, and it motivated me to write this book to share both my professional knowledge and personal insights with the hope of making the menopausal journey a bit smoother for women everywhere.

As I write this book, I draw from my experiences as a pharmacist and as a woman who has walked the path of menopause. I understand the challenges, but I also appreciate the opportunities for growth, self-discovery, and empowerment that it can bring. My personal story has not only deepened my connection with the women I serve but also provided a unique perspective that I hope will resonate with and support my readers on their respective journeys through menopause.

Why a Pharmacist's Perspective Matters in Menopause

A pharmacist's perspective is significant in menopause for several compelling reasons.

Medication expertise: Pharmacists are experts in medications, including hormone replacement therapy (HRT) and other drugs commonly prescribed during menopause. They can provide valuable guidance on the appropriate use of these medications, potential side effects, drug interactions, and dosage adjustments.

Accessibility: Pharmacists are often more accessible than doctors, making them a valuable resource for women seeking information and advice about managing menopausal symptoms. Women can visit their local pharmacies and consult with a pharmacist without an appointment.

Over-the-counter (OTC) recommendations: Pharmacists can recommend OTC products and supplements that can help alleviate common menopausal symptoms. They guide in selecting the right products and ensure their safety and efficacy.

Drug interactions: Menopausal women may be taking multiple medications for various health conditions. Pharmacists can assess potential drug interactions and advice on managing medications safely to prevent adverse effects.

Customized solutions: Every woman's experience with menopause is unique. Pharmacists can tailor their recommendations to the specific needs and preferences of individual women, providing personalized solutions to address their symptoms.

Patient education: Pharmacists are skilled communicators and can explain complex medical information in a way that is easy for patients to understand. They can educate women about the physical and hormonal changes that occur during menopause and the impact of medications on their health.

Wellness promotion: Pharmacists offer holistic guidance on maintaining overall health during menopause. They can advise on nutrition, exercise, sleep, and mental health strategies, promoting a well-rounded approach to menopausal wellness.

Trust and accessibility: Many women have long-standing relationships with their pharmacists and trust them as healthcare providers. This trust makes it easier for women to discuss personal and sensitive topics related to menopause.

Collaboration with healthcare providers: Pharmacists can collaborate with doctors and other healthcare providers to ensure that women receive comprehensive care during menopause. This inter-professional approach helps to address the diverse needs of menopausal women.

Continuous learning: Pharmacists are committed to continuous learning and staying up-to-date with the latest research and guidelines. This ensures that they provide women with the most current and evidence-based information on menopause management.

In summary, a pharmacist's perspective is crucial in menopause because they bring expertise in medications, accessibility, and the ability to provide personalized solutions. Their role in educating, guiding, and collaborating with healthcare providers makes them a vital part of the support network for women going through this significant life transition.

A Journey through Menopause: Setting the Stage for a Fulfilling Journey

Welcome to this remarkable and transforming journey through menopause. In this introduction, we set the stage for the profound importance of this life transition and the essential reasons for embarking on this journey with purpose and empowerment.

Embracing the inevitability

Menopause, dear reader, is a reality - a shared facet of the female experience. It signifies the conclusion of their reproductive years and the initiation of a new and exciting chapter. As we venture into this exploration, it is essential for women to embrace this inevitability, for only in doing so can we truly understand and navigate it with grace and assurance.

The menopausal spectrum

Menopause is not a singular event but rather a multi-faceted spectrum encompassing perimenopause, menopause itself, and postmenopause; each characterized by its unique attributes and hurdles. By delving into the distinctions between these stages, we pave the way for a more comprehensive grasp of what awaits you.

Knowledge as empowerment

Knowledge is a source of unparalleled empowerment. The wisdom you gain throughout this journey will be your guiding light. In the chapters to come, we will furnish you with indispensable insights into the physical, emotional, and psychological facets of menopause. Armed with this knowledge, you will be equipped to make informed choices about your health and well-being.

Building a supportive community

Though every woman's experience with menopause is distinct, a profound sense of solidarity unites us all. This introduction emphasizes the significance of fostering a community of understanding and mutual support. The stories and experiences we share will fortify the camaraderie that underlies this journey, serving as a wellspring of strength and encouragement.

Anticipating the future

Menopause is not a culmination but a vibrant new beginning. It heralds a chance to prioritize your well-being, discover new passions, and greet the changes brought with wisdom and maturity. This introduction sets the stage for you to look ahead, to relish the possibilities that menopause unveils, and to cultivate a positive outlook for the adventure that lies ahead.

As we embark on this voyage together, remember that your menopausal journey can be a rewarding, spirited, and enriching one. By understanding the various stages, seeking knowledge, and embracing the support and solidarity of a community of fellow travelers, you can traverse this path with confidence and anticipation. Menopause is not a conclusion; instead, it is a captivating new chapter in your remarkable life.

CHAPTER 1:MENOPAUSE BASICS

Understanding the Science and Physiology behind Menopause

Menopause, a critical stage in a woman's life, is defined by the cessation of menstruation and the accompanying hormonal changes. It is a natural biological process that typically occurs to women in their late 40s to early 50s. It marks the end of a woman's reproductive years. It is crucial to comprehend the science and physiology behind this transformative transition in order to embark on a fulfilling journey through menopause.

The role of hormones

Hormones are at the heart of menopause. During a woman's reproductive years, the ovaries produce estrogen and progesterone, which regulate the menstrual cycle and fertility. As menopause approaches, these hormone levels begin to fluctuate and decline. This hormonal shift is responsible for many of the symptoms and changes associated with menopause.

The ovarian reserve

A fundamental aspect of menopause is the concept of ovarian reserve. A woman is born with a finite number of eggs, and this reserve steadily diminishes over time. As the number of eggs declines, the ovaries become less responsive to hormonal signals from the brain. This process triggers the characteristic changes associated with menopause.

Perimenopause: The transition phase

Menopause is not an abrupt event but a gradual process. The years leading up to menopause are known as perimenopause. During this transition phase, hormonal fluctuations can cause irregular menstrual cycles and a variety of symptoms, such as hot flashes, mood swings, and sleep disturbances. Understanding perimenopause is essential because it is often the time when women seek support and interventions to manage their symptoms.

The impact of menopause on reproductive health

Menopause signifies the end of a woman's reproductive capability. While fertility significantly declines during perimenopause, the potential for pregnancy still exists until a woman has gone 12 consecutive months without a menstrual period. Women need to be well informed about their reproductive health and options during this phase.

Bodily changes

Beyond the cessation of menstruation, menopause can lead to various physical changes. These include a decrease in bone density, an increased risk of heart disease, and changes in body composition. It is important to understand how these changes affect overall health and what preventive measures can be taken.

By grasping the science and physiology behind menopause, women can gain insights into the biological underpinnings of this natural transition. This knowledge empowers women to make informed decisions about their health, explore treatment options, and embark on their menopausal journey with confidence and understanding. In the chapters to come, we will delve deeper into the specific aspects of menopause, from its hormonal intricacies to the management of its diverse symptoms, offering a comprehensive guide to navigating this transformative stage of life.

Differentiating between Perimenopause, Menopause, and Postmenopause

In the journey through menopause, we encounter distinct phases that shape this transformative process. Let's explore these phases in a more fluid narrative:

Perimenopause: A prelude to change

Perimenopause is the prelude to menopause, a transitional phase that usually starts in a woman's 40s. It is a time when the body begins to undergo significant changes in preparation for menopause. Critical characteristics of perimenopause include:

- **Irregular menstrual cycles**: You may notice changes in the regularity and flow of your periods. In some months, your cycle may be longer or shorter than usual.
- **Hormonal fluctuations**: Hormone levels, especially estrogen, start to fluctuate. This can lead to symptoms like hot flashes, mood swings, and sleep disturbances.
- **Ovulation changes**: Ovulation becomes irregular, affecting fertility. Contraception is necessary if you do not wish to conceive.
- **Symptoms of onset of menopause**: Perimenopause is when many women begin to experience menopausal symptoms, such as hot flashes and night sweats.

Menopause: The Transformation

Menopause is the central event in this journey. It is the point when a woman has not menstruated for 12 consecutive months. While the average age of menopause is around 51, it can occur between the late 40s and early 50s. Critical characteristics of menopause include:

- **Cessation of menstruation**: When menstrual periods cease, it is a clear indication of the transition into menopause.

•   **Hormonal changes**: Hormone levels, particularly estrogen and progesterone, significantly decrease, leading to various physical and emotional symptoms.

•   **Common symptoms**: Menopausal symptoms, such as hot flashes, night sweats, mood swings, and vaginal dryness, become more pronounced.

•   **Reduced fertility**: Women are no longer fertile during menopause, although pregnancy remains possible in the months leading up to it.

Postmenopause: The Continuation of Your Journey

Postmenopause follows menopause and continues throughout the rest of your life. Its defining features are:

•   **Stabilized hormone levels**: Hormone levels, especially estrogen, stabilize at lower levels during postmenopause. The most severe hormonal fluctuations and symptoms that occur during perimenopause and menopause become less pronounced.

•   **Higher risk of certain health conditions**: The risk of conditions such as osteoporosis and heart disease may increase during postmenopause due to the ongoing effects of reduced estrogen.

•   **Continuation of certain symptoms**: Although many menopausal symptoms decrease in intensity, some, like vaginal dryness and changes in sexual health, can persist and may require ongoing management.

•   **Health maintenance**: Maintaining overall health becomes paramount during postmenopause. Regular medical check-ups, appropriate lifestyle adjustments, and a focus on bone health, heart health, and mental well-being are essential.

This journey through perimenopause, menopause, and postmenopause is a dynamic and transformative process. Understanding the phases, their characteristics, and implications empowers you to navigate this transition with grace and knowledge, ensuring a fulfilling and vibrant life beyond menopause.

CHAPTER 2: THE ROLE OF HORMONES IN MENOPAUSE

Exploring Hormonal Changes and Their Impact on Menopause

Hormonal changes are at the core of menopause, and these changes have a profound impact on a woman's body and overall health. The hormonal changes that occur during menopause and their effects are enumerated below:

- **Decline in estrogen:** Estrogen, the primary female sex hormone, plays a central role in the menstrual cycle and various bodily functions. During menopause, estrogen levels gradually decline, leading to several effects:

  - *Hot flashes:* The decrease in estrogen levels can disrupt the body's temperature regulation, leading to hot flashes, which are sudden and intense sensations of heat, often accompanied by sweating and flushing.
  - *Vaginal changes:* Estrogen helps maintain the thickness and elasticity of the vaginal lining. With declining estrogen levels, the vaginal tissues become thinner, drier, and less elastic,

leading to symptoms like vaginal dryness and pain during intercourse.

- *Bone health*: Estrogen is essential for maintaining bone density. Its decline can lead to a loss of bone mass and increase the risk of osteoporosis, a condition characterized by brittle and fragile bones.
- *Mood and cognitive changes:* Estrogen also influences mood and cognitive function. Some women may experience mood swings, irritability, or memory issues during menopause.

- **Decline in progesterone:** Progesterone, another female sex hormone, helps regulate the menstrual cycle. In menopause, progesterone levels also decrease, which can result in:

- *Irregular or absent periods:* The hormonal imbalance caused by low progesterone can lead to erratic menstrual cycles and eventually to the absence of periods.
- *Elevated follicle-stimulating hormone (FSH):* As estrogen levels decrease, the pituitary gland increases the production of FSH. Elevated FSH levels are a hallmark of menopause and are used to diagnose it. FSH plays a role in stimulating the ovaries to produce eggs and is involved in the regulation of estrogen.

- *Vasomotor symptoms:* FSH, in combination with declining estrogen, contributes to vasomotor symptoms, such as hot flashes and night sweats.

- **Other hormonal changes:** Menopause also involves changes in other hormones, such as testosterone. Testosterone levels can decrease as women age, and this may impact sexual desire and energy levels.

The impact of these hormonal changes during menopause can vary widely from one woman to another. Some women may experience only mild symptoms, while others may have more severe and disruptive effects on their quality of life. Genetic factors, lifestyle, and overall health can influence the symptoms and their intensity.

Managing the hormonal changes and their impact

•   **Hormone replacement therapy (HRT)**: HRT involves replacing the declining hormones, primarily estrogen and sometimes progesterone. This can effectively alleviate many of the symptoms associated with menopause but should be carefully considered due to potential risks and benefits.

- **Lifestyle changes:** A healthy diet, regular exercise, and stress management can help alleviate some of the symptoms and promote overall well-being during menopause.

- **Non-Hormonal medications:** Some women opt for non-hormonal medications or complementary therapies to manage specific symptoms, such as antidepressants for mood swings or lubricants for vaginal dryness.
- **Regular health check-ups:** Women in menopause should have regular check-ups with their healthcare providers to monitor bone density, cardiovascular health, and other aspects of their well-being.

Understanding the hormonal changes and their impact on menopause is crucial for women to make informed decisions about how to manage this natural phase of life and to maintain their health and quality of life as they age. Consulting with a healthcare provider is essential to tailor an approach that suits an individual's unique needs and health considerations.

Pros and Cons of Hormone Replacement Therapy (HRT)

Hormone Replacement Therapy (HRT) can be a valuable treatment option for some individuals, primarily women going through menopause; however, it also comes with both potential benefits and risks. It is essential to weigh the pros and cons in consultation with a healthcare provider to determine if HRT is a suitable choice for an individual's specific situation.

Pros of Hormone Replacement Therapy (HRT)

Relief from menopausal symptoms: HRT can effectively alleviate a range of menopausal symptoms, including hot flashes, night sweats, vaginal dryness, and mood swings, improving a woman's overall quality of life.

Bone health: Estrogen replacement can help maintain bone density and reduce the risk of osteoporosis, a condition characterized by brittle bones prone to fractures.

Cardiovascular benefits: Some studies suggest that HRT might have cardiovascular benefits, including a reduction in the risk of heart disease when started early in the menopausal transition. However, this is a subject of ongoing research and debate.

Improved skin and hair: Estrogen can help improve skin elasticity and thickness, as well as maintain the quality of hair.

Prevention of vaginal atrophy: HRT can prevent or alleviate vaginal atrophy; which is characterized by thinning and dryness of vaginal tissues, making sexual activity more comfortable.

Cons of Hormone Replacement Therapy (HRT)

Health risks: HRT is associated with potential health risks. The Women's Health Initiative (WHI) study found an increased risk of specific health issues among postmenopausal women using HRT, including an elevated risk of blood clots, stroke, and breast cancer. The risks can vary based on the type of HRT (estrogen-only or combination therapy), duration of use, and an individual's health history.

Breast cancer risk: The use of HRT, particularly combination therapy (estrogen plus progestin), is associated with a slightly increased risk of breast cancer. The risk is generally higher with long-term use.

Cardiovascular risks: While some studies suggest the cardiovascular benefits of HRT, others have raised concerns about the increased risk of blood clots, stroke, and heart disease. These risks may vary depending on the timing of HRT initiation and an individual's cardiovascular health.

Not suitable for everyone: HRT may not be appropriate for women with a history of certain medical conditions, such as breast cancer, heart disease, or a history of blood clots.

Side effects: Like any other medication, HRT can have side effects, including breast tenderness, bloating, headaches, and mood changes.

Cost and convenience: HRT can be costly, and it often requires regular doctor visits for monitoring and prescription renewals.

Individual variation: The effectiveness and tolerance of HRT can vary widely among individuals, so it may not provide relief from symptoms for everyone.

It is important to emphasize that the decision to use HRT should be individualized and made in consultation with a healthcare provider. They can help assess the potential benefits and risks based on an individual's medical history, age, and menopausal symptoms. Some women may choose to use HRT for a limited time to manage severe menopausal symptoms. In contrast, others may opt for alternative approaches, such as lifestyle changes and non-hormonal therapies. Regular follow-up and re-evaluation of the treatment plan are also essential to adjust or discontinue HRT as needed.

CHAPTER 3: COMMON MENOPAUSAL SYMPTOMS

Hot Flashes, Night Sweats, Mood Swings, and Other Symptoms

Let us take an in-depth look at each of these symptoms:

Hot flashes (Hot flushes)

Description: Hot flashes are sudden and intense sensations of heat that usually start in the upper body and can spread to the face, neck, and sometimes the entire body. They are often accompanied by sweating, flushing, and a rapid heartbeat.

Frequency and Duration: Hot flashes can vary in frequency and duration. They typically last for a few minutes but can occur multiple times a day.

Cause: Hot flashes are primarily attributed to the hormonal changes of menopause, particularly the decrease in estrogen levels. The exact mechanisms behind hot flashes are not fully understood.

Night sweats

Description: Night sweats are episodes of extreme sweating during sleep, which can drench the bedclothes and lead to disrupted sleep.

Frequency and Duration: Night sweats often coincide with hot flashes, and they can lead to poor sleep quality, fatigue, and irritability.

Cause: Night sweats are essentially hot flashes that occur during sleep. They result from hormonal changes, particularly the drop in estrogen levels. They can be exacerbated by factors such as room temperature and bedding.

Mood swings

Description:Mood swings refer to rapid and often unpredictable changes in mood, including irritability, anxiety, sadness, and sometimes even anger.

Frequency and Duration: Mood swings can be episodic and vary in intensity. They can affect a woman's emotional well-being.

Cause: The hormonal fluctuations during menopause, especially the drop in estrogen, can affect neurotransmitters in the brain. Hormonal imbalances can contribute to mood swings and emotional changes. Psychological factors, lifestyle changes, and stress can also play a role.

Irregular periods

Description: As women approach menopause, their menstrual cycles become irregular. This means that periods may occur more or less frequently and can be lighter or heavier than usual.

Frequency and Duration: Irregular periods can persist for several years during the menopausal transition.

*Cause:*Irregular periods are a direct result of hormonal changes. The ovaries become less responsive to hormonal signals from the brain, leading to unpredictable ovulation and menstruation.

Vaginal changes

*Description:*Vaginal changes include thinning and drying of vaginal tissues, which can lead to symptoms like vaginal dryness, itching, pain during intercourse, and an increased risk of vaginal infections.

*Frequency and duration:*These changes typically become more pronounced as menopause progresses and may persist beyond menopause.

*Cause:*Decreased estrogen levels lead to changes in the vaginal lining and reduced lubrication. This can impact sexual comfort and overall vaginal health.

Difficulty sleeping

*Description:*Many women going through menopause experience sleep disturbances, including difficulty falling asleep, staying asleep, or experiencing night sweats that disrupt their sleep.

Frequency and duration: Sleep problems can persist throughout the menopausal transition.

Cause: Hormonal changes, night sweats, and psychological factors can contribute to sleep difficulties.

Management and Alleviation of these Symptoms using Pharmaceutical and Non-pharmaceutical Approaches

Managing and alleviating menopausal symptoms involves a combination of pharmaceutical and non-pharmaceutical approaches tailored to an individual's specific needs and preferences. Here are strategies for addressing common menopausal symptoms:

1. Hot flashes and night sweats

Pharmaceutical approaches:

- **Hormone replacement therapy (HRT):** For severe symptoms, HRT can be highly effective. It involves the use of estrogen alone or in combination with progestin (for women with a uterus). Consult with a healthcare provider to assess the risks and benefits of HRT based on your medical history.
- **Prescription medications:** Non-hormonal prescription medications, such as selective serotonin reuptake inhibitors (SSRIs) and serotonin-norepinephrine reuptake inhibitors (SNRIs), can help reduce the frequency and intensity of hot flashes and night sweats.

Non-Pharmaceutical Approaches

- **Lifestyle modifications:** Avoiding triggers like spicy foods, caffeine, and alcohol may help. Dressing in layers and using portable fans can provide quick relief during hot flashes.
- **Cooling strategies:** Keep your sleeping environment cool, use moisture-wicking bedding, and consider cooling pillows.
- **Relaxation techniques:** Techniques like deep breathing, yoga, and meditation can help manage stress and reduce the frequency and severity of hot flashes.

2. Mood swings

Pharmaceutical approaches

For mood swings and emotional changes, medication may not always be necessary. However, for women experiencing severe mood disturbances, antidepressants or anti-anxiety medications may be considered. Consult a healthcare provider for guidance.

Non-Pharmaceutical Approaches

- **Counseling or therapy:** Psychotherapy, such as cognitive-behavioral therapy, can help manage mood swings and emotional changes.
- **Regular exercise**: Physical activity can improve mood and reduce anxiety and depression.
- **Stress reduction:** Stress management techniques, like mindfulness and relaxation exercises, can be effective in managing mood swings.

3. Irregular periods

Pharmaceutical approaches

If irregular periods are bothersome or associated with heavy bleeding, HRT or non-hormonal medications, such as nonsteroidal anti-inflammatory drugs (NSAIDs) or tranexamic acid, can be considered.

Non-pharmaceutical approaches

- **Healthy diet:** Eating a balanced diet rich in fruits, vegetables, and whole grains can support hormonal balance.
- **Regular exercise:** Maintaining a healthy weight and engaging in regular physical activity can help regulate periods.
- **Stress management:** Reducing stress through relaxation techniques can help regulate the menstrual cycle.

4. Vaginal changes

Pharmaccutical approaches

- **Vaginal Estrogen:** Low-dose vaginal estrogen therapy, in the form of creams, rings, or tablets, can effectively treat vaginal dryness and discomfort. It delivers estrogen directly to the vaginal tissues with minimal systemic absorption.

Non-pharmaceutical approaches

- **Water-based lubricants:** Over-the-counter water-based lubricants can provide temporary relief during intercourse.
- **Regular sexual activity:** Engaging in regular sexual activity can help maintain vaginal health and reduce discomfort.

5. Difficulty sleeping

Pharmaceutical approaches

- For sleep disturbances, short-term use of medications, such as hypnotics or sleep aids, may be considered. Consult with a healthcare provider before using sleep medications.

Non-pharmaceutical approaches:

- **Sleep hygiene:** Develop healthy sleep habits, such as keeping a consistent sleep schedule, creating a comfortable sleep environment, and avoiding caffeine and screens before bedtime.
- **Relaxation techniques:** Relaxation exercises, such as progressive muscle relaxation or meditation, can promote better sleep.

It is essential to consult with your doctor before starting any pharmaceutical treatment, especially hormone replacement therapy, as it involves risks and benefits that vary among individuals. Additionally, a healthcare provider can help tailor a comprehensive approach that combines both pharmaceutical and non-pharmaceutical strategies to manage menopausal symptoms effectively. Regular follow-up is crucial to monitor the effectiveness and adjust the treatment plan as needed.

CHAPTER 4:MEDICATIONS AND SUPPLEMENTS

Overview of Pharmaceutical and Non-prescription Options for Symptoms Management

Menopause can lead to a variety of physical and emotional symptoms, and women may seek both pharmaceutical and non-prescription options for symptom management. Here is an overview of some common approaches:

Pharmaceutical options

- **Hormone replacement therapy (HRT):** HRT is the most effective treatment for relieving the symptoms of menopause. It involves taking estrogen, often in combination with progestin (for women with a uterus), to replace the hormones that are declining during menopause. HRT can be administered in various forms, including pills, patches, gels, creams, and vaginal rings. However, HRT is not suitable for everyone, and its use should be carefully considered and discussed with a healthcare provider due to potential risks and benefits.

- **Selective serotonin reuptake inhibitors (SSRIs)**: Some antidepressant medications, like fluoxetine and paroxetine, can help manage hot flashes and mood swings in menopausal women.
- **Gabapentin and pregabalin:** These medications, which are often used to treat seizures and nerve pain, can also help reduce hot flashes.
- **Clonidine:** Normally used to treat high blood pressure, clonidine can help alleviate hot flashes in some women.
- **Ospemifene and conjugated estrogens/bazedoxifene:** These are non-hormonal prescription medications approved to treat moderate to severe vaginal dryness and painful intercourse associated with menopause.

Non-prescription options

- **Lifestyle Modifications:** Healthy lifestyle choices can help alleviate menopausal symptoms. These include maintaining a balanced diet, regular exercise, and managing stress. Avoiding caffeine, alcohol, and spicy foods may reduce the frequency and intensity of hot flashes.
- **Phytoestrogens:** Found in foods like soy, flaxseed, and red clover; phytoestrogens are plant compounds that mimic estrogen in the body. Some women find relief from symptoms by increasing their intake of these foods.
- **Herbal supplements:** Herbal remedies like black cohosh and evening primrose oil are sometimes used to alleviate hot flashes, though their effectiveness is still debated.
- **Vaginal lubricants and moisturizers:** Over-the-counter products like lubricants and moisturizers can help alleviate vaginal dryness and discomfort.
- **Cooling products:** Cooling pillows, clothing, and fans can provide relief for hot flashes.

- **Mind-Body Techniques:** Practices such as yoga, meditation, and deep breathing exercises can help manage stress, mood swings, and sleep disturbances associated with menopause.
- **Acupuncture:** Some women find acupuncture to be effective in reducing hot flashes and improving sleep.

It is essential to consult with your healthcare provider before starting any medication or supplement regimen, especially if you have underlying health conditions. The choice of treatment should be based on an individual's specific symptoms, medical history, and preferences. Healthcare professionals can help women make informed decisions regarding the most appropriate approach to managing menopausal symptoms.

Potential Drug Interactions and Side Effects

Pharmaceutical options for managing menopausal symptoms, such as hormone replacement therapy (HRT) and prescription medications can have potential drug interactions and side effects that women should be aware of. It's crucial to consult with a healthcare provider before starting any medication to understand these risks and benefits as individual responses can vary. Here's an overview of potential drug interactions and common side effects associated with these treatments:

Hormone replacement therapy (HRT)

Potential drug interactions:

- **Blood thinners:** Estrogen can interact with blood-thinning medications like warfarin, potentially increasing the risk of bleeding.
- **Anticonvulsants:** Some anticonvulsant drugs, such as phenytoin and carbamazepine, may reduce the effectiveness of HRT.

- **Certain antibiotics:** Some antibiotics can reduce estrogen absorption, potentially reducing the effectiveness of HRT.
- **St. John's Wort:** This herbal supplement may decrease the effectiveness of estrogen in HRT.

Common side effects:

- **Breast tenderness:** Some women may experience breast tenderness or enlargement.
- **Nausea:** HRT can cause nausea or stomach discomfort, especially when taken orally.
- **Vaginal bleeding:** Irregular vaginal bleeding is a common side effect, particularly in the first few months of HRT.
- **Fluid retention:** Some women may experience mild fluid retention or weight gain.
- **Headaches:** Headaches can occur as a side effect of HRT.
- **Mood changes:** Mood swings or changes in mood are possible side effects.
- **Increased risk of blood clots and stroke:** HRT can increase the risk of blood clots and stroke, especially in women with certain risk factors.

Prescription Medications for Menopausal Symptoms

The specific drug interactions and side effects can vary depending on the medication, but here are some general considerations:

Potential drug interactions:

- **SSRIs and SNRIs:** Potential interactions with other medications can occur when using antidepressants like SSRIs and SNRIs for mood swings. Always consult a healthcare provider about potential interactions with other medications you may be taking.
- **Gabapentin and Pregabalin:** These medications can interact with other drugs, so it's important to inform your healthcare provider of all medications you're using.

Common side effects:

- **Nausea:** Nausea can be a common side effect of some medications.
- **Dizziness:** Dizziness or lightheadedness can occur with certain medications.
- **Dry mouth:** Dry mouth can be a side effect of some medications.
- **Digestive issues:** Some medications can cause digestive problems such as constipation or diarrhea.
- **Sleep disturbances:** Changes in sleep patterns may occur with certain drugs.
- **Weight changes:** Weight gain or loss can be a side effect of some medications.

It's important to remember that individual responses to medications can vary. Your healthcare provider will take into account your medical history and any potential drug interactions when prescribing these treatments. They will also closely monitor your response and adjust the treatment plan as needed.

Additionally, discuss the benefits and risks of treatment thoroughly with your healthcare provider, especially regarding the potential long-term risks associated with HRT, such as an increased risk of certain cancers, blood clots, and cardiovascular disease. Women should make informed decisions regarding their treatment based on individual health and symptoms.

CHAPTER 5: WOMEN'S HEALTH AND MENOPAUSE

Addressing Bone Health and Osteoporosis During and After Menopause

Addressing bone health and osteoporosis during and after menopause is crucial because the hormonal changes associated with menopause can lead to bone loss and an increased risk of fractures. Here are some key strategies to promote and maintain bone health during this period:

- **Calcium and vitamin D intake:**

Adequate calcium intake is essential for maintaining bone density. Postmenopausal women should aim for 1,200-1,500mg of calcium daily through dietary sources and supplements, if necessary.

Vitamin D is essential for calcium absorption and bone health. Ensure adequate exposure to sunlight, or consider Vitamin D supplements.

- **Balanced diet:**

Consume a diet rich in fruits, vegetables, lean proteins, and whole grains to provide essential nutrients for bone health.

Limit excessive consumption of salt, caffeine, and alcohol, as they can contribute to bone loss.

- **Weight-bearing exercises:**

Engage in weight-bearing exercises such as walking, jogging, dancing, and resistance training to help maintain bone density and muscle strength.

- **Bone density testing:**

Regular bone density tests (DEXA scans) are recommended to assess bone health and the risk of osteoporosis. The frequency of testing may vary based on individual risk factors.

Medications for osteoporosis

If bone density tests show significant bone loss or if you have a high risk of osteoporosis, your healthcare provider may prescribe medications such as bisphosphonates, denosumab, or hormone therapy to prevent further bone loss.

Lifestyle modifications:

- Quit smoking, as it can contribute to bone loss.
- Limit alcohol consumption to reduce the risk of osteoporosis.
- Minimize the risk of falls by keeping homes safe and well-lit, using handrails, and wearing appropriate footwear.

Hormone replacement therapy (HRT):
Hormone replacement therapy (HRT) can have a positive impact on bone density. However, the decision to use HRT should be made carefully, considering both the benefits and potential risks, as discussed with a healthcare provider.

Evaluate risk factors:
Assess individual risk factors, including family history, personal medical history, and lifestyle choices. Discuss these factors with your healthcare provider to determine your risk of osteoporosis.

Consider bisphosphonate therapy:
Bisphosphonates are a class of medications that help slow bone loss and reduce the risk of fractures. Your healthcare provider may recommend them if you have a significant risk of osteoporosis.

Fall prevention:

Preventing falls is essential to avoid fractures. This includes maintaining good balance, using assistive devices if necessary, and ensuring that your home environment is safe.

Regular follow-up with healthcare provider:
Regular check-ups with your healthcare provider are essential to monitor bone health, assess the effectiveness of treatments, and make necessary adjustments to your plan.

It is important to remember that bone health is a lifelong process. The steps taken during and after menopause can significantly affect bone density and fracture risk. Consult with a healthcare provider to develop a personalized plan that addresses your specific needs and risk factors for osteoporosis.

Cardiovascular Health Considerations for Women in Midlife

Maintaining cardiovascular health is a critical concern for women in midlife and beyond, particularly during the menopausal transition. Several factors, including hormonal changes, age-related issues, and lifestyle choices, can influence heart health. Here are key considerations on how to support cardiovascular well-being.

Understanding risk factors

Women should begin by recognizing individual risk factors for heart disease. Common risk factors include high blood pressure, high cholesterol, diabetes, a family history of heart disease, smoking, obesity, and physical inactivity.

Diet for heart health

Adopting a heart-healthy diet is essential. This entails reducing the intake of saturated and trans fats, cholesterol, and sodium while prioritizing fruits, vegetables, whole grains, lean proteins, and heart-healthy fats from sources like nuts and olive oil. Processed foods and sugary beverages should be limited.

Weight management

Maintaining a healthy weight is vital for heart health. Achieving this goal typically requires a combination of a nutritious diet and regular physical activity.

Regular exercise

Engaging in routine physical activity is crucial. Strive for at least 150 minutes of moderate-intensity aerobic exercise or 75 minutes of vigorous-intensity aerobic exercise each week. It's also beneficial to incorporate strength training exercises to preserve muscle mass and boost metabolism.

Blood pressure care

Monitor and manage blood pressure regularly. Hypertension is a significant risk factor for heart disease. If prescribed medication, follow the regimen as directed.

Cholesterol control

Regularly check cholesterol levels and work with healthcare providers to address high cholesterol through lifestyle changes or medication, if necessary.

Diabetes management

For those with diabetes, effectively managing blood sugar levels is essential, as elevated blood sugar can damage blood vessels and increase heart disease risk.

Smoking Cessation

Quitting smoking is critical for heart health. Smoking is a significant contributor to heart disease.

Moderate alcohol consumption

Consume alcohol in moderation, if you must. Excessive alcohol intake can contribute to heart problems.

Stress reduction

Chronic stress can negatively affect heart health. Engage in stress-reduction techniques like mindfulness, meditation, and relaxation exercises.

Hormone replacement therapy (HRT) considerations

If contemplating hormone replacement therapy (HRT) to manage menopausal symptoms, discuss the potential benefits and risks with a healthcare provider. HRT may have both positive and negative effects on heart health, and the decision should be individualized.

Regular health check-ups

Routine check-ups with healthcare providers are essential for monitoring cardiovascular health. These appointments typically include blood pressure checks, cholesterol level assessments, and evaluations of overall heart function.

Awareness of heart attack symptoms

Women should familiarize themselves with the warning signs of a heart attack. While chest pain or discomfort is a common symptom, women may also experience shortness of breath, nausea, lightheadedness, and pain in the neck, jaw, or back. Recognizing these symptoms is crucial for seeking prompt medical attention.

In summary, taking proactive steps to support cardiovascular health is paramount for women in midlife and beyond. Regular check-ups, a heart-healthy lifestyle, and an awareness of heart disease risk factors can significantly reduce the likelihood of heart-related issues. Heart disease is a leading cause of mortality among women, and early prevention and management are crucial to maintaining a healthy heart throughout midlife and beyond.

CHAPTER 6:MENTAL AND EMOTIONAL WELL-BEING

Navigating the Emotional Challenges that can Accompany Menopause

Navigating the emotional challenges that can accompany menopause is a vital aspect of this life transition. Menopause, characterized by hormonal changes and the cessation of menstruation, can bring about a range of emotional symptoms. Here's how to manage these challenges effectively:

Education and understanding

Start by educating yourself about menopause. Understanding the physical and emotional changes associated with this transition can help you prepare and reduce anxiety.

Seek support

Share your experiences and emotions with friends, family, or a support group. Talking to others who are going through or have gone through menopause can provide validation and comfort.

Communicate with your partner

Discuss your feelings and experiences with your partner. Open and honest communication can strengthen your relationship during this time.

Self-care

Prioritize self-care, including adequate sleep, regular exercise, and a balanced diet. These practices can help improve mood and reduce stress.

Stress reduction techniques

Explore stress reduction techniques like mindfulness, meditation, yoga, or deep breathing exercises. These can help you manage anxiety and emotional ups and downs.

Therapy or counseling

Consider therapy or counseling, especially if you're struggling with severe emotional symptoms. A mental health professional can offer guidance and support.

Hormone replacement therapy (HRT)

For some women, HRT may help alleviate emotional symptoms associated with menopause. Discuss the potential benefits and risks of HRT with a healthcare provider.

Herbal and alternative remedies

Some women find relief from emotional symptoms with the use of herbal remedies like black cohosh or dietary supplements such as Omega-3 fatty acids. Consult a healthcare provider before using any alternative therapies.

Acceptance and self-compassion

Understand that emotional changes are a natural part of menopause. Be kind to yourself and allow yourself to feel and express your emotions without judgment.

Manage lifestyle factors

Identify lifestyle factors that may contribute to emotional challenges. These could include an unhealthy diet, lack of exercise, or excessive stress. Make necessary adjustments.

Maintain an active social life

Continue to engage in social activities and maintain a supportive network of friends. Social connections can be a source of emotional support.

Set realistic expectations

Recognize that menopause is a significant life transition, and it's okay to take things at your own pace. Set realistic expectations for yourself and understand that it is a process.

Seek professional help for severe symptoms

If you experience severe emotional symptoms like depression or severe anxiety, consult a mental health professional or psychiatrist. Treatment options, including therapy and medication, may be necessary.

Navigating the emotional challenges of menopause is a personal journey, and it's important to remember that not every woman will experience the same emotional symptoms. By seeking support, practicing self-care, and being open to different treatment options, you can better manage the emotional challenges that may arise during this natural phase of life.

Strategies for Maintaining Mental Health and Well-being

Maintaining mental health and well-being is an ongoing journey, and it's crucial during significant life transitions like menopause. As you navigate this phase, consider the following strategies to support your mental health and overall well-being:

- **Self-compassion:** Approach this period with self-compassion. Menopause is a natural part of life, and it's okay to have mixed feelings about it. Be kind to yourself, acknowledge your emotions, and avoid self-criticism.
- **Education and awareness:** Educate yourself about menopause and its potential impact on mental health. Understanding the physical and emotional changes that can occur will help you feel more in control and less anxious.
- **Seek support:** Don't hesitate to share your experiences and emotions with friends, family, or a support group. Talking to others who are going through or have gone through menopause can provide validation and comfort.
- **Communication with loved ones:** Engage in open and honest conversations with your partner and loved ones about what you're going through. Their support can be priceless during this transition.
- **Self-care:** Prioritize self-care, including getting enough sleep, maintaining a balanced diet, and engaging in regular physical activity. Self-care is the foundation of mental well-being.
- **Stress reduction:** Explore stress-reduction techniques such as mindfulness, meditation, yoga, or deep breathing exercises. These practices can help you manage anxiety and emotional fluctuations.
- **Emotional expression:** Permit yourself to express your emotions, whether through journaling, creative outlets, or simply talking to a trusted friend. Bottling up emotions can lead to greater distress.
- **Professional help:** If you find that your emotional symptoms are severe or significantly impacting your daily life, consider

seeking therapy or counseling from a mental health professional. Therapy can provide tools and strategies to cope with emotional challenges.

- **Hormone replacement therapy** (HRT): If deemed suitable, discuss the potential benefits and risks of hormone replacement therapy (HRT) with a healthcare provider. HRT can have an impact on both physical and emotional menopausal symptoms.
- **Regular check-ups:** Maintain regular health check-ups, including discussions about your mental health, with a healthcare provider. They can provide guidance and monitor any changes in your well-being.
- **Purpose and engagement:** Continue to engage in activities that bring you joy and a sense of purpose. Pursue hobbies, interests, or volunteer work that provides a sense of fulfillment.
- **Social connections:** Maintain and nurture your social connections. Strong social support can help buffer the emotional challenges of menopause.
- **Acceptance and adaptation:** Remember that menopause is a natural phase of life. Embrace it as an opportunity for personal growth and self-discovery. Adapt to the changes it brings and find new ways to thrive.
- **Professional guidance for severe symptoms:** If you experience severe emotional symptoms such as depression or severe anxiety, consult a mental health professional or psychiatrist. Treatment options, including therapy and medication, may be necessary.

These strategies can be integrated into your daily life as you journey through menopause and beyond. Remember that everyone's experience is unique, and it's essential to tailor your approach to what works best for you. By nurturing your mental health and overall well-being, you can make this transition a period of personal growth and self-discovery.

CHAPTER 7:NUTRITION AND MENOPAUSE

How Dietary Choices Can Impact Menopausal Symptoms and Overall Health

Dietary choices significantly influence menopausal symptoms and overall health. Menopause, marked by hormonal changes, can be better managed and even eased through proper nutrition. Here's how dietary choices can make a difference:

- Manage menopausal symptoms: Diet plays a role in managing various menopausal symptoms:
- Hot flushes:Reducing the intake of spicy foods, caffeine, and alcohol can help alleviate hot flashes.
- Mood swings: Nutrient-rich foods, particularly complex carbohydrates found in whole grains, fruits, and vegetables can stabilize blood sugar levels and improve mood swings.
- Vaginal dryness:Foods rich in healthy fats, like fatty fish, nuts, and seeds, can support vaginal health by promoting natural lubrication.
- Bone health:Menopausal hormonal changes can lead to reduced bone density. A diet rich in Calcium and Vitamin D is crucial. Sources include dairy products, leafy greens, fortified plant-based milk, and sunlight exposure.

- Heart health:Heart disease risk increases post-menopause. A heart-healthy diet emphasizes fruits, vegetables, whole grains, lean proteins, and healthy fats like olive oil and nuts. Reducing saturated fats and processed foods can lower cholesterol levels and support heart health.
- Weight management:Menopausal hormonal changes may lead to weight gain. A balanced diet featuring whole foods, lean proteins, and high-fiber options can help with weight management.
- Gut health: Menopause can impact gut health. A diet rich in fiber from fruits, vegetables, and whole grains can promote a healthy gut microbiome.
- Blood pressure: Maintaining healthy blood pressure is essential for heart health. Reducing sodium intake by avoiding high-sodium processed foods can help.
- Hormone balance: Phytoestrogens in soy, flaxseeds, and legumes may help balance hormones during menopause.
- Hydration: Adequate water intake is vital for managing symptoms like dry skin and vaginal dryness and is essential for overall health.
- Antioxidants: Foods rich in antioxidants, such as berries, dark leafy greens, and colorful fruits and vegetables, combat oxidative stress and inflammation associated with aging and menopause.
- Protein: Adequate protein supports muscle health, which can decline with age. Include lean protein sources like poultry, fish, lean meats, and plant-based options like tofu and legumes.
- Processed foods: Minimizing processed foods high in sugar, unhealthy fats, and preservatives, helps prevent symptoms exacerbation and weight gain. Prioritize whole, unprocessed foods.
- Dietary supplements: Depending on individual needs, dietary supplements such as Calcium, Vitamin D, and Omega-3 fatty acids may be beneficial. Consult with a healthcare provider before adding supplements.

- Portioncontrol:Be mindful of portion sizes to prevent overeating and weight gain, particularly as metabolism slows down with age.

Dietary choices have a profound impact on managing menopausal symptoms and overall well-being. A balanced, nutrient-rich diet tailored to individual symptoms and nutritional needs can help women better navigate the challenges of menopause and promote long-term health.

Special Considerations for Maintaining a Healthy Diet During this Life Phase

Maintaining a healthy diet during the menopausal phase requires a thoughtful approach due to the significant changes happening in a woman's body. Here are some key factors to consider when planning your diet during menopause:

- Hormonal changes: Menopause introduces hormonal fluctuations that can affect metabolism and fat storage, potentially leading to weight gain, particularly around the abdominal area. To support weight management, focus on portion control and whole foods while you minimize processed and high-sugar items.
- Bone health: Hormonal shifts during menopause increase the risk of osteoporosis and reduced bone density. Ensure sufficient intake of Calcium and Vitamin D to support bone health, including sources like dairy products, fortified plant-based milk, leafy greens, and sunlight for Vitamin D.
- Heart health: Post-menopause, the risk of heart disease rises. Prioritize a heart-healthy diet by including fruits, vegetables, whole grains, lean proteins, and healthy fats like olive oil, nuts, and fatty fish. Reduce saturated fats and processed foods.
- Menopausal symptoms:Diet can influence menopausal symptoms. To manage hot flashes, reduce intake of spicy foods, caffeine, and alcohol. Mood swings may benefit from complex carbohydrates found in whole grains, fruits, and

vegetables. For vaginal health and dryness reduction, incorporate healthy fats from nuts and seeds.

- Gut health:Menopause can impact gut health, so a diet rich in fiber from sources like fruits, vegetables, and whole grains can promote a healthy gut microbiome.
- Hydration:Stay well hydrated as it's crucial for managing symptoms like dry skin and vaginal dryness, and it supports overall health.
- Hormone balance: Foods containing phytoestrogens, such as soy, flaxseeds, and legumes, have estrogen-like properties that may help balance hormones during menopause.
- Antioxidants: An antioxidant-rich diet with berries, dark leafy greens, and colorful fruits and vegetables can combat oxidative stress and inflammation associated with aging and menopause.
- Protein:Adequate protein intake supports muscle health, which is essential as muscle mass tends to decline with age. Choose lean protein sources like poultry, fish, lean meats, tofu, and legumes.
- Processed foods: Minimize processed foods high in sugar, unhealthy fats, and preservatives, as they can exacerbate symptoms and lead to weight gain. Opt for whole, unprocessed foods whenever possible.
- Dietary supplements: Depending on individual needs and any potential deficiencies, dietary supplements like Calcium, Vitamin D, and Omega-3 fatty acids may be beneficial. Consult with a healthcare provider before adding supplements to your diet.
- Portion control: Keep an eye on portion sizes to prevent overeating and weight gain, particularly as metabolism tends to slow down with age.

Adapting your diet with these special considerations can help you manage menopausal symptoms and promote overall health. Individual experiences vary, so working with a healthcare provider or nutritionist to create a personalized dietary plan is a wise choice during this life phase.

CHAPTER 8:EXERCISE AND PHYSICAL WELLNESS

The Role of Physical Activity in Alleviating Menopausal Symptoms

Physical activity plays a significant role in alleviating menopausal symptoms. Menopause, a natural stage in a woman's life, brings various physical and psychological challenges, including hot flashes, mood swings, weight gain, and decreased bone density. Engaging in regular physical activity can help mitigate these symptoms:

- **Hot flashes and night sweats**: Hot flashes and night sweats are common and bothersome menopausal symptoms. Regular exercise can help regulate body temperature and improve overall circulation, potentially reducing the frequency and intensity of these episodes.
- **Mood swings and depression:** Hormonal fluctuations associated with menopause can lead to mood swings and depression. Physical activity stimulates the release of endorphins, natural mood lifters, and helps reduce stress and anxiety, promoting mental well-being.

- **Weight management:** Many women experience weight gain during menopause due to a decrease in metabolism and changes in fat distribution. Regular exercise can help prevent weight gain by increasing metabolism, building muscle, and promoting a healthy body composition.
- **Bone health:** Menopause is associated with a decline in bone density, increasing the risk of osteoporosis. Weight-bearing exercises like walking, running, and resistance training help strengthen bones and reduce this risk.
- **Heart health:** Menopause can impact heart health due to decreased estrogen levels. Regular physical activity, especially aerobic exercises, can help maintain cardiovascular health by lowering blood pressure and cholesterol levels.
- **Sleep quality:** Many women experience sleep disturbances during menopause. Regular exercise can improve sleep quality by regulating sleep patterns and reducing insomnia.
- **Cognitive function:** Some research suggests that physical activity may have a positive impact on cognitive function and memory during menopause.

It's crucial to customize the type, intensity, and frequency of exercise to individual needs and fitness levels. Consulting with a healthcare professional or fitness expert is advisable for creating a personalized exercise plan. Additionally, combining physical activity with a balanced diet and other lifestyle changes enhances the management of menopausal symptoms.

In summary, physical activity is a valuable tool for managing the symptoms of menopause. It can improve physical and mental well-being, alleviate hot flashes, support weight management, promote bone and heart health, and contribute to better sleep and cognitive function during this transitional phase in a woman's life.

Tailored Exercise Routines and Approaches for Women in Menopause

Tailored exercise routines and approaches for women in menopause are essential to address the unique physical and hormonal changes they experience during this life stage. Here are some guidelines for creating personalized exercise plans for women in menopause:

- **Consultation with a healthcare professional**

Before starting any exercise routine, women in menopause should consult with a healthcare professional, such as a gynecologist or primary care physician, to ensure they are physically ready for exercise. This is particularly important if there are underlying health conditions.

- **Assess current fitness level**

A baseline assessment of current fitness and physical abilities is crucial. This can include tests for strength, flexibility, cardiovascular fitness, and bone density.

- **Set realistic goals**

Work with a fitness professional to set achievable goals based on individual needs and preferences. Goals may include weight management, improved mood, better sleep, increased bone density, or enhanced cardiovascular health.

- **Balanced exercise routine**

A well-rounded exercise plan should include a combination of aerobic, strength training, and flexibility exercises. Here's how to incorporate them:

- *Aerobic exercise*: Engage in activities like walking, cycling, swimming, or dancing to improve cardiovascular health. Aim for at least 150 minutes of moderate-intensity aerobic exercise per week.

- *Strength training:* Incorporate resistance exercises, such as weight lifting, bodyweight exercises, or resistance bands, to build and maintain muscle mass. Strength training should be done at least two days a week.

- *Flexibility and balanced exercises:* Include yoga, Pilates, or stretching routines to maintain flexibility and balance, which can be especially important as women age.

- *Adapt to individual preferences:* Exercise routines should align with individual preferences and lifestyles. Some women may prefer group fitness classes, while others may enjoy solitary activities. The key is to choose activities that are enjoyable and sustainable.

- **Modify intensity and duration**

As hormonal changes can affect energy levels and recovery, it's essential to listen to the body. Modify the intensity and duration of workouts as needed, especially during days of increased fatigue or menopausal symptoms.

- **Focus on bone health**

Weight-bearing exercises like walking and strength training are crucial for maintaining bone density and reducing the risk of osteoporosis. Ensure these are part of the routine.

- **Consider core muscle strengthening**

Strengthening the core muscles can help alleviate lower back pain and improve posture, which can be particularly relevant during menopause.

- **Monitor menopausal symptoms**

Keep track of how exercise affects menopausal symptoms. For instance, some women may find that aerobic exercise helps reduce hot flashes. In contrast, others may benefit more from relaxation techniques.

- **Stay hydrated and wear appropriate clothing**

Due to the increased risk of overheating and dehydration during menopause, it's essential to stay hydrated and wear appropriate workout attire.

- **Progressive overload**

Progressive overload essentially means pushing your body beyond its current capabilities in a systematic way. For example, if you're lifting weights, you might increase the weight you lift as your strength improves. If you're doing bodyweight exercises, you could increase the number of repetitions or sets.

This principle is crucial because as your body adapts to a certain level of stress, it becomes more efficient, and the initial gains might slow down. By gradually increasing the workload, you consistently challenge your body, promoting muscle growth, strength development, and overall fitness improvements. It's a key strategy to avoid hitting a plateau and keep making progress in your fitness journey.

- **Rest and recovery**

Ensure that adequate rest and recovery periods are included in the exercise plan to prevent overtraining and injuries.

- **Mind-body practices**

Incorporate stress-reduction techniques like mindfulness, meditation, or tai chi to manage mood swings and reduce stress and anxiety.

- **Regular Health Check-Ups**

Continue with regular health check-ups to monitor overall health and address any specific concerns related to menopause.

Remember that every woman's experience of menopause is unique, so it's essential to create a tailored exercise plan that considers individual needs, goals, and preferences. A fitness professional or personal trainer with experience in menopause-related fitness can provide valuable guidance and support in designing and adjusting the exercise routine as needed.

CHAPTER 9:SLEEP AND MENOPAUSE

Addressing Sleep Disturbances and Strategies for Improving Sleep Quality

Addressing sleep disturbances and improving sleep quality is crucial for overall well-being, particularly during menopause when hormonal changes can disrupt sleep patterns. Here are some strategies to help women in menopause manage sleep disturbances and improve the quality of their sleep:

- **Establish a consistent sleep schedule**

Try to go to bed and wake up at the same time every day, even on weekends. This helps regulate your body's internal clock and can improve the quality of your sleep.

- **Create a relaxing bedtime routine**

Engage in calming activities before bedtime, such as reading, taking a warm bath, or practicing relaxation techniques like deep breathing or meditation. These activities can signal to your body that it's time to wind down.

- **Limit exposure to screens**

Avoid using electronic devices such as smartphones, tablets, or computers for at least an hour before bedtime. The blue light emitted from screens can disrupt your body's production of melatonin, a hormone that regulates sleep.

- **Watch your diet**

Be mindful of what you eat and drink in the evening. Avoid large meals, caffeine, and alcohol close to bedtime, as they can interfere with sleep. Opt for a light, healthy snack if needed.

- **Create a comfortable sleep environment**

Ensure your bedroom is conducive to sleep. Keep the room cool, dark, and quiet. Consider using blackout curtains, earplugs, or a white noise machine if necessary.

- **Invest in a comfortable mattress and pillow**

A quality mattress and pillow that provide adequate support can make a significant difference in sleep comfort.

An orthopedic mattress, designed to offer optimal support for the spine and joints, is a great example. Its focus on providing proper alignment can contribute to improved sleep quality, especially during the challenges of menopause.

- **Regular exercise**

Engaging in regular physical activity can improve sleep quality. Aim for at least 30 minutes of moderate-intensity exercise most days of the week, but avoid vigorous exercise too close to bedtime.

- **Manage stress and anxiety**

Stress and anxiety can be expected during menopause and can interfere with sleep. Practice stress-reduction techniques like yoga, meditation, or progressive muscle relaxation to help calm the mind.

- **Manage hot flashes**

If hot flashes are disrupting your sleep, try keeping the bedroom cooler and wearing lightweight, breathable sleepwear. Some women find that relaxation techniques can help reduce the frequency and intensity of hot flashes.

- **Hormone replacement therapy (HRT)**

In some cases, hormone replacement therapy prescribed by a healthcare provider can help manage menopausal symptoms, including sleep disturbances. Discuss the potential benefits and risks with your healthcare professional.

- **Consult a sleep specialist**

If sleep problems persist despite trying these strategies, consider consulting a sleep specialist or a healthcare provider who can help diagnose and treat underlying sleep disorders.

- **Limit naps**

While short daytime naps can be refreshing, long or irregular napping during the day can disrupt nighttime sleep. If you need to nap, keep it brief (20-30 minutes) and earlier in the day.

- **Cognitive behavioral therapy for insomnia (CBT-I)**

CBT-I is a structured program that helps individuals identify and replace thoughts and behaviors that cause or worsen sleep problems. It can be an effective treatment for sleep disturbances during menopause.

Improving sleep quality during menopause may require a combination of lifestyle changes and, in some cases, medical intervention. It's essential to be patient and persistent in finding what works best for you. Consulting with a healthcare professional or sleep specialist can provide further guidance and solutions for addressing sleep disturbances and promoting restful sleep.

Pharmaceutical and Non-pharmaceutical Approaches to Managing Sleep Issues

Managing sleep issues can involve both pharmaceutical and non-pharmaceutical approaches. The choice between these options should be made in consultation with a healthcare provider, taking into consideration the specific causes and severity of the sleep problems. Here's an overview of pharmaceutical and non-pharmaceutical approaches to managing sleep issues:

Non-pharmaceutical approaches

❖ **Lifestyle Modifications**

- *Sleep Hygiene:* Establishing good sleep hygiene practices, such as maintaining a consistent sleep schedule, creating a comfortable sleep environment, and avoiding stimulating activities before bedtime.
- *Diet and Exercise:* Maintaining a healthy diet and engaging in regular physical activity can promote better sleep. Avoiding heavy meals and caffeine close to bedtime is advisable.
- *Cognitive-Behavioral Therapy for Insomnia (CBT-I):* This structured therapy focuses on identifying and changing behaviors and thought patterns that contribute to insomnia. It is effective for improving sleep without medication.

❖ **Relaxation techniques:**

- *Mindfulness meditation:* Practicing mindfulness meditation can help reduce stress and promote relaxation before bedtime.
- *Progressive muscle relaxation*: A technique involving tensing and relaxing muscle groups to reduce physical tension and anxiety.

- *Stress management:* Reducing stress through techniques like deep breathing exercises, yoga, or tai chi can improve sleep quality.

❖ **Natural supplements**

Some individuals find relief from sleep issues with supplements like melatonin, valerian root, or chamomile. However, it's essential to consult with a healthcare provider before using any supplements, as they may interact with other medications or have side effects.

❖ **Light therapy**

Light therapy, especially for those with circadian rhythm disorders, involves exposure to bright light during specific times of the day to regulate the sleep-wake cycle.

Pharmaceutical approaches

- Prescription of Sleep Medications: In cases of severe and chronic sleep disturbances, healthcare providers may prescribe medications, such as:

- **Benzodiazepines:** These are sedative medications that can help induce sleep.
- **Non-benzodiazepine hypnotics:** These are newer sleep medications with a lower risk of dependence compared to benzodiazepines.
- **Melatonin receptor agonists:** These medications, like ramelteon, act on the body's melatonin receptors to regulate sleep-wake cycles.
- **Sedating antidepressants:** Certain antidepressant medications, such as trazodone, are sometimes prescribed off-label for their soothing effects.
- **Hormone therapy:** In some cases, hormone replacement therapy (HRT) can be prescribed to address sleep disturbances related to hormonal imbalances, such as those experienced during menopause.

- **Antihistamines:** Over-the-counter antihistamines, like diphenhydramine, can have sedating effects and are occasionally used to induce sleep.
- **Other medications:** In some situations, medications designed for other purposes, such as antipsychotics or antiepileptic drugs, may be prescribed off-label to address sleep issues. However, this should be under the guidance of a healthcare provider.

Pharmaceutical approaches should be considered when non-pharmaceutical methods have been unsuccessful or when sleep issues are severe, persistent, or significantly influencing quality of life. A healthcare provider, taking into account potential side effects, interactions, and individual needs should carefully consider the choice of medication and its duration.

Additionally, combining non-pharmaceutical and pharmaceutical approaches can often be an effective strategy for managing sleep issues, as this allows individuals to address the root causes of their sleep problems while providing short-term relief when needed.

CHAPTER 10:SEXUAL HEALTH AND INTIMACY

Changes in Sexuality and Intimacy During Menopause

Menopause triggers a range of changes in sexuality and intimacy for women. These transformations stem from hormonal shifts, physical symptoms, and psychological factors, and they can vary widely from one individual to another. Here's an overview of the usual shifts that women may experience during menopause:

- **Decreased libido:** Many women notice a decline in sexual desire (libido) as estrogen levels decrease during menopause. This can affect their sexual arousal and desire.
- **Vaginal dryness:** Reduced estrogen levels can lead to vaginal dryness and thinning of the vaginal walls, making sexual intercourse uncomfortable or painful, which can impact sexual enjoyment.
- **Changes in sexual response:** Hormonal changes during menopause may cause alterations in sexual response, including decreased genital sensitivity and difficulties reaching orgasm.

- **Mood swings and stress:** Menopause often brings mood swings, irritability, and increased stress, which can affect a woman's emotional well-being and her ability to engage in intimate relationships.
- **Hot flashes and night sweats:** The discomfort of hot flashes and night sweats can disrupt sleep and overall comfort, potentially reducing interest in sexual activity.
- **Body image concerns:** Changes in body composition, such as weight gain, can affect self-esteem and body image, potentially impacting sexual confidence and intimacy.
- **Fatigue:** Sleep disturbances and hormonal fluctuations can lead to fatigue, reducing the desire or ability to engage in sexual activity.
- **Relationship dynamics:** Menopause can also influence relationship dynamics. Effective communication with a partner becomes crucial as couples navigate these changes together.

Despite these challenges, it is important to note that menopause can also bring positive changes and opportunities for women:

- **Increased self-confidence:** Some women report feeling more self-confident and empowered during menopause, which can positively affect their approach to sexuality and intimacy.
- **Freedom from contraception:** With the cessation of menstruation, women no longer need to worry about contraception, which can reduce some stress and make intimacy more relaxed.
- **Focus on emotional connection:** As hormonal changes may affect sexual response, couples may place a greater emphasis on emotional intimacy and communication.
- **Exploration and adaptation:** Some women and their partners use menopause as an opportunity to explore new sexual experiences and adapt to the changes in their bodies and desires.

To address changes in sexuality and intimacy during menopause, women and their partners can consider various strategies:

- **Open and honest communication:** Discussing concerns, desires, and needs with a partner can help maintain a solid emotional connection.
- **Medical consultation:** Seeking advice from a healthcare provider can address specific issues such as vaginal dryness or discomfort during intercourse.
- **Lubrication and moisturizers:** Over-the-counter or prescription products can help alleviate vaginal dryness.
- **Behavioral and psychological approaches:** Engaging in stress-reduction techniques, counseling, or therapy can help manage mood swings and improve emotional well-being.
- **Experimentation and adaptation:** Couples can explore different sexual activities and communication methods to adapt to changing desires and needs.

It's crucial to remember that every woman's experience of menopause is unique. What works for one person may not work for another, so an individualized approach is crucial to maintaining a satisfying and fulfilling intimate life during and after menopause.

Strategies to Maintain a Fulfilling Sexual Life During this Phase

Maintaining a fulfilling sexual life during various phases of life, including menopause, often requires adjustments and strategies to address physical and emotional changes. Here are some strategies for women and their partners to consider:

- **Open communication:** Effective communication with your partner is essential. Discuss your desires, concerns, and needs openly. This can help both partners understand each other better and foster a deeper emotional connection.
- **Education:** Understanding the physical and emotional changes that come with menopause can help alleviate anxiety and misunderstandings. Seek reputable sources of information and books, or attend educational workshops together.

- **Medical consultation:** If specific issues like vaginal dryness, pain during intercourse, or other sexual health concerns are affecting your intimacy, consult a healthcare provider. They can provide guidance and recommend treatments or therapies, such as hormone replacement therapy (HRT) or topical treatments for vaginal dryness.
- **Mindfulness and relaxation:** Engage in mindfulness practices, meditation, or relaxation techniques to reduce stress and anxiety, improving emotional well-being and potentially enhancing intimacy.
- **Prioritize emotional connection:** During menopause, emotional intimacy can become more critical than ever. Focus on nurturing your emotional connection through shared activities, quality time together, and meaningful conversations.
- **Experiment and adapt:** Be open to trying new things in the bedroom. As desires and physical responses may change, being open to experimentation can be exciting and satisfying.
- **Lubrication and moisturizers:** Over-the-counter or prescription lubricants and moisturizers can help alleviate vaginal dryness and discomfort during intercourse, making the experience more comfortable.
- **Counseling and therapy:** Individual or couple's counseling or therapy can provide a safe space to discuss intimate issues, improve communication, and address emotional concerns.
- **Kegel exercises:** These exercises can help strengthen the pelvic floor muscles, improving sexual response and potentially reducing issues like urinary incontinence. Consult with a healthcare provider or a physical therapist for guidance on these exercises.
- **Natural supplements:** Some women find relief from sexual issues through natural supplements like black cohosh, ginseng, or ginkgo biloba. Please consult with a healthcare provider before using any supplements to ensure they are safe and appropriate for your situation.
- **Sexual well-being products:** Explore sexual well-being products designed to enhance intimacy, such as arousal gels,

toys, or erotic literature, if both partners are comfortable with them.

- **Scheduled intimacy:** Setting aside specific times for intimacy can help ensure that you prioritize your sexual life, even when other aspects of life are busy.
- **Stay physically active:** Regular exercise can boost your mood, improve self-esteem, and increase overall well-being. It can also have a positive impact on sexual desire and satisfaction.
- **Healthy lifestyle choices:** Eating a balanced diet, managing stress, and getting enough rest can contribute to better overall health, which can, in turn, positively impact your sexual life.

Remember that maintaining a fulfilling sexual life during menopause is about adapting to changes, focusing on the emotional connection, and exploring new ways to experience intimacy. Every woman's experience is unique, and it's important to prioritize what feels suitable for you and your partner. Consulting with healthcare professionals or sexual health experts can provide additional guidance and support.

CHAPTER 11:PERSONAL GROWTH AND RESILIENCE

How to Embrace Menopause as an Opportunity for Personal Growth

Embracing menopause as an opportunity for personal growth is a transformative mindset that can empower women during this life transition. Here are practical steps and insights to help women see menopause as a chance for personal development:

- **Shift your perspective:** Menopause is a natural phase of life, not an ending. Begin by reframing your perspective. See it as a chapter of growth and self-discovery, just like any other life stage.
- **Self-reflection:** Take time to reflect on your life journey. Consider the experiences, challenges, and achievements that have shaped you. Menopause is an ideal time to reconnect with your past and celebrate your resilience.
- **Body positivity:** Embrace the physical changes that come with menopause. Love and appreciate your body for its strength and the stories it carries. Accepting your changing physique can boost self-esteem.

- **Mind-body connection:** Recognize the powerful connection between your thoughts and physical well-being. Positive thinking can influence how you experience menopause and impact your overall health.
- **Wisdom and experience:** Menopause is a period of profound wisdom and experience. Recognize the knowledge and insights you've gained throughout your life. This wisdom can guide and inspire you.
- **Reevaluate priorities:** Use menopause as an opportunity to reassess your life's priorities. What dreams and aspirations have you postponed? It's time to revive them and pursue what truly matters to you.
- **Emotional growth:** Menopause can bring emotional challenges; mood swings and irritability are common. Understand that these emotions are a natural part of the journey and can lead to emotional growth and resilience.
- **Holistic health:** Prioritize your overall health and wellness. Proper nutrition, regular exercise, and self-care are essential to feeling your best during menopause.
- **Strengthen relationships:** Focus on strengthening your relationships, especially with your partner. Open communication, emotional support, and understanding can bring you closer.
- **New beginnings:** See menopause as a new beginning. Just as each day brings new opportunities, menopause can usher in a fresh phase of life filled with renewed energy and enthusiasm.
- **Community and support:** Connect with like-minded individuals who are experiencing menopause. Joining support groups or online forums can provide valuable insights and a sense of community.
- **Personal goals and challenges:** Set new personal goals and challenges. Whether it is pursuing a new career, embarking on a creative project, or exploring a new hobby, personal growth is an ongoing process.
- **Reconnect with yourself:** Invest time in self-reflection and self-discovery. Reconnect with your core values and passions.

Menopause can be a time to embrace a more authentic version of yourself.

- **A gift of transformation:** Ultimately, recognize menopause as a gift of transformation. It's an opportunity to celebrate the journey, savor the wisdom, and step into the future with enthusiasm and grace.

Embracing menopause as an opportunity for personal growth is a journey of self-acceptance, self-care, and self-discovery. It's a chance to celebrate the uniqueness of this phase and unlock the potential for personal development and empowerment.

Stories of Women Who Have Thrived During and After Menopause

I wish to share a few stories with you here of some amazing women who have thrived during and after menopause for inspiration and motivation. These real-life accounts demonstrate that menopause is not a hindrance but a transformative phase that can lead to personal growth and empowerment. Let me start with my own story:

** I am a Pharmacist in my late 50s, and I just discovered in me this new talent of putting pen to paper. Here I am, writing books and enjoying it. It is quite fulfilling. I am making my little contributions to the literary world at this particular stage in my life.*

- **Susan's journey of self-discovery**

Susan, a successful businesswoman, used menopause as an opportunity to explore her creative side. She began painting and found immense joy in the process. Over time, she transitioned into a successful artist and discovered a new, fulfilling career.

- **Maria's health and fitness transformation**

After experiencing menopause, Maria decided to take control of her health and well-being. She started a regular exercise routine, embraced a healthier diet, and lost weight. Her newfound vitality not only improved her physical health but also boosted her self-esteem and confidence.

- **Rebecca's rekindled passion for travel**

Rebecca had always dreamt of traveling the world, but the responsibilities of her younger years kept her grounded. In menopause, she decided it was time to make her dream a reality. She started by taking solo trips and eventually created a travel blog that inspired other women to pursue their travel dreams.

- **Aisha's late-career success**

Aisha, in her late 50s, decided to change her career path during menopause. She went back to school, pursued a degree in a field she was passionate about, and started her own consulting business. Her story demonstrates that there is always time to chase your professional dreams.

- **Jennifer's thriving relationship**

Menopause brought new challenges to Jennifer's marriage, but she and her husband decided to face them together. They attended couples' counseling and used the transition as an opportunity to deepen their emotional connection. Their relationship thrived, and they found new ways to enjoy their time together.

- **Saratu's volunteer work**

After retiring from her long-term job, Saratu sought a sense of purpose during menopause. She became a dedicated volunteer at a local nonprofit organization, using her skills to make a difference in her community. This involvement brought her a profound sense of fulfillment.

- **Carol's entrepreneurial spirit**

Carol's entrepreneurial journey started during menopause. She identified a gap in the market for natural menopause relief products and founded her own company. Her story illustrates how menopause can be a catalyst for innovation and business success.

- **Amina's adventure in education**

Amina, a mother of three, decided to go back to school during menopause to complete her degree. Despite the challenges, she graduated and became a teacher. Her story shows that learning and personal growth can continue at any age.

These real-life stories illustrate the diverse ways women have thrived during and after menopause. They serve as a reminder that menopause can be a catalyst for personal growth, self-discovery, and the pursuit of dreams. I hope these narratives will inspire and empower you to embrace menopause as a transformative opportunity in your lives.

CHAPTER 12: THE ROLE OF THE PHARMACIST

The Pharmacist's Role in Helping Women Navigate Menopause

Menopause can be a bumpy journey; but fear not, for in the midst of this transformative storm, your pharmacist stands as a steadfast lighthouse, guiding you through the tumultuous seas.

Understanding menopause

Before we delve into the pharmacist's role, let us try to understand what menopause truly means. It is not merely the cessation of menstruation; rather, it is a profound shift in your body's hormonal landscape. Your pharmacist, armed with knowledge and compassion, will help you navigate these changes. They will explain the intricate dance of hormones and the stages leading up to menopause, giving you the roadmap you need to sail through this transition.

The pharmacist's role in menopause care

The pharmacist is your trusted navigator on this voyage. In the world of healthcare, they are often underestimated, but their role in menopause care is pivotal. They offer more than just pills and potions; they provide patient-centered care. Your pharmacist listens to your concerns, answers your questions, and offers a personalized approach to managing your menopausal symptoms. They're your confidant, providing not just medications but also invaluable support.

Over-the-counter (OTC) products and supplements

You have probably heard about over-the-counter products and supplements that promise relief from hot flashes and sleepless nights. However, your pharmacist separates fact from fiction. They help you navigate the aisles, guiding you to products that are not only effective but also safe. Before you reach for that bottle, you can trust your pharmacist to offer expert advice.

Hormone replacement therapy (HRT)

Hormone Replacement Therapy, or HRT, is a significant aspect of menopause management. It's a complex topic with potential benefits and risks. Your pharmacist doesn't just dispense HRT; they are your source of wisdom. They will explain the pros and cons, help you choose the right option, and monitor your progress. With their guidance, you can make informed decisions about your health.

Lifestyle and nutrition

Menopause isn't just about medications; it's a holistic journey. Your pharmacist understands the importance of lifestyle and nutrition. They act as your health coach, offering guidance on diet and exercise, helping you embrace a healthier lifestyle to navigate this transition with grace.

Emotional well-being

Emotions can run wild during menopause. Your pharmacist acknowledges the mood swings and the emotional turbulence. They offer not just medications but also a listening ear. They guide you toward counseling or support groups because they know that emotional well-being is just as vital as physical health.

Sexual health

Intimacy is a crucial aspect of life, and menopause can affect it. Your pharmacist addresses the changes in vaginal health and suggests solutions. They foster open conversations about relationships and communication because they understand that a healthy sex life is part of your overall well-being.

Staying informed and advocating for your health

Empowerment is the key. Your pharmacist encourages you to stay informed, to ask questions, and to advocate for your health. They are your partner in this journey, reminding you to have regular check-ups and ensuring you discuss your menopause-related concerns with healthcare professionals.

Embrace menopause with confidence, for your pharmacist is more than just a dispenser of medications but also your beacon of knowledge, guide to better health, and unwavering support system. With their expertise and empathy, you can navigate the uncharted waters of menopause with grace and strength. The pharmacist's role is instrumental, and together, you will conquer this transformative journey.

Tips for Effectively Communicating with Healthcare Providers

Effective communication with healthcare providers is crucial for menopausal women to receive the best care and support during this significant life transition. Here are some tips to help women communicate effectively with their healthcare providers:

- **Prepare in advance:** Before your appointment, make a list of questions and concerns you want to discuss. Jot down your symptoms, their frequency, and any triggers you've noticed.

- **Be open and honest:** Share all your symptoms and concerns, even if they seem minor or embarrassing. Healthcare providers are there to help, and nothing is too trivial to mention.
- Be honest about any lifestyle factors, such as smoking, alcohol use, or changes in your diet, as these can influence your menopausal experience.

- **Keep a symptom diary:** Maintain a diary of your symptoms, including when they occur and any pattern you notice. This can help your healthcare provider better understand your situation.
- **Discuss your menstrual history:** Provide information about your menstrual history, including the age at which you started your period, the regularity of your cycles, and when your last period occurred. This information is essential for diagnosing menopause.
- **Ask questions:** Feel free to ask questions if you need help understanding something your healthcare provider has said. Request clarification until you're confident in your understanding.
- **Seek clarification:** If your healthcare provider recommends a specific treatment or therapy, ask for a clear explanation of the benefits, risks, and potential side effects. Make sure you understand your options.
- **Discuss your treatment preferences:** Express your preferences regarding treatment options. Some women may prefer non-hormonal therapies, while others may be open to hormone replacement therapy (HRT).
- **Bring a trusted companion:** If you feel overwhelmed during appointments or anticipate that you might need to remember

important information, bring a trusted friend or family member with you to provide support and help you remember what was discussed.

- **Be specific and descriptive:** When discussing symptoms, be specific and descriptive. Instead of saying, *"I feel bad,"* explain what you are experiencing, such as, *"I have hot flashes multiple times a day, and they disrupt my sleep."*
- **Discuss emotional and psychological health:** Menopause can have a significant impact on emotional well-being. Be open about any mood change, anxiety, or depression you may be experiencing.
- **Explore alternative therapies:** If you are interested in complementary or alternative therapies, ask your healthcare provider for their opinion and any potential benefits or risks.
- **Follow up:** After your appointment, follow up with your healthcare provider if you have any concern or if your symptoms change. Regular communication ensures that your treatment plan can be adjusted as needed.
- **Advocate for yourself:** Remember that you are your best advocate. If you feel that your concerns need to be addressed or that your treatment isn't effective, feel free to seek a second opinion or explore other healthcare providers.

Effective communication is essential for receiving personalized care and making informed decisions about managing menopausal symptoms. Your healthcare provider is there to support you, and by being open and proactive, you can work together to navigate this significant life transition with confidence.

CHAPTER 13:EMPOWERING YOURSELF

Advocating for Your Health and Well-being during Menopause

Menopause is a unique and transformative phase in a woman's life, marking the end of the reproductive years and the beginning of a new chapter. While it is a natural transition, the symptoms and changes that come with menopause can be challenging. To navigate this journey successfully and ensure you receive the care and support you deserve, it is essential to become an advocate for your health and well-being. Here's how:

- ***Know your body:*** It is important to understand the stages of menopause and how they can affect your body. Knowledge is empowering, and being informed about what is happening to your body is the first step in advocacy.
- ***Open Communication:*** Establish an open line of communication with your healthcare provider. Share your concerns, symptoms, and goals. Ask questions and be an active participant in your healthcare decisions.

- ***Research and Information:*** Educate yourself about menopause, treatment options, and lifestyle changes that can help alleviate symptoms. Knowledge enables you to make informed choices.
- ***Create a Support System:*** Seek support from friends and family who understand your experience. Share your journey with them, and let them be part of your support system.
- ***Set Personal Goals:*** Define your health and well-being goals during menopause; whether it's managing specific symptoms, staying active, or embracing a healthier lifestyle, set clear objectives.
- ***Embrace Lifestyle Changes:*** Incorporate healthy habits into your daily routine. Focus on a balanced diet, regular exercise, stress management, and adequate sleep.
- ***Treatment Options:*** Discuss treatment options with your healthcare provider, including hormone therapy, non-hormonal treatments, or alternative therapies. Make decisions based on what aligns best with your goals and values.
- ***Monitor Your Progress:*** Keep track of how your symptoms are changing and whether your chosen treatment is effective. Regularly update your healthcare provider on your progress.
- ***Emotional Well-being:*** Address the emotional aspects of menopause. Seek counseling or support groups if needed. Your emotional health is just as important as your physical health.
- ***Advocate for Equal Treatment:*** If you feel your concerns aren't taken seriously, or your symptoms are being dismissed, be assertive in advocating for the care you deserve.
- ***Second Opinions:*** Feel free to seek a second opinion if you feel your current healthcare provider needs to meet your needs. Your health is a priority, and it's crucial to find the proper support.
- ***Share Your Experience:*** Share your menopause journey with others. By speaking openly about your experience, you can help reduce the stigma around menopause and encourage other women to advocate for their health.

Menopause is a unique journey for every woman, and advocating for your health and well-being is an essential part of that journey. By taking an active role in your healthcare and embracing a healthy lifestyle, you can navigate menopause with confidence and ensure that this transition is a positive and empowering phase of your life. Remember, you are your best advocate, and your health and well-being are worth it.

Resources for Further Information, Support, and Self-Empowerment

Books:

- **"The Wisdom of Menopause"** by Dr. Christiane Northrup: A comprehensive guide to understanding menopause and embracing it as a transformative phase.
- **"Menopause Confidential"** by Dr. Tara Allmen: Provides practical advice and evidence-based information to empower women during menopause.
- **"The Menopause Book"** by Barbara Kantrowitz and Pat Wingert: A thorough exploration of menopause with insights from medical experts.

Websites:

- North American Menopause Society (NAMS) - The NAMS website offers a wealth of resources, including articles, webinars, and a directory of menopause healthcare providers.
- Women's Health - The official website of the U.S. Department of Health & Human Services provides information on women's health, including menopause.
- Menopause Matters - A UK-based website with articles, forums, and a directory of healthcare professionals specializing in menopause.

Support groups:

Joining local or online menopause support groups can provide a sense of community and a safe space to share experiences and advice with other women going through the same journey—websites like Inspire and HealthUnlocked host various health-related forums, including menopause discussions.

Healthcare providers:

Your healthcare provider is a valuable resource for personalized advice and treatment options during menopause. Feel free to ask questions and discuss your concerns.

Mobile apps:

There are mobile apps available that can help you track your menopausal symptoms, provide information, and offer tips for managing them. Examples include "Menopause Pal" and "MenoPro".

Counseling and therapy:

Consider seeking counseling or therapy if you're experiencing emotional challenges during menopause. A qualified mental health professional can provide support and coping strategies.

Hormone therapy clinics:

If you are considering hormone replacement therapy (HRT), consult with a hormone therapy specialist who can provide expert guidance and personalized treatment options.

Alternative and complementary medicine practitioners:

If you're interested in alternative therapies, such as acupuncture or herbal remedies, consult with experienced practitioners who specialize in menopausal care.

Wellness and fitness programs:

Many fitness centers and wellness studios offer programs tailored to menopausal women. These can include exercise classes, nutrition counseling, and stress-reduction techniques.

Podcasts and webinars:

Many podcasts and webinars focus on women's health and menopause. These can provide expert insights, personal stories, and valuable tips for managing menopausal symptoms.

Remember that your experience of menopause is unique, and it's important to find resources and support that align with your specific needs and preferences. Empowering yourself with knowledge and connecting with others who understand what you're going through can make this transition smoother and more positive.

CHAPTER 14:CONCLUSION

A Summary of Key Points from This Book

"Navigating Menopause: Your Essential Guide to a Life in Full Bloom" is an uplifting and informative resource that equips women with the knowledge and tools to embrace the transformative phase of menopause. The book emphasizes the importance of viewing this natural life transition as an opportunity for personal growth and newfound freedom.

Key takeaways from this guide include:

Embracing change: Menopause is a positive journey of self-discovery and personal growth.

Comprehensive knowledge: The book offers a wealth of information about the physical, emotional, and psychological aspects of menopause, empowering women to understand their bodies and minds during this phase.

Wellness strategies: Practical advice is provided for managing common menopausal symptoms, such as hot flashes, mood swings, and sleep disturbances. It also covers tips on nutrition, exercise, and holistic approaches for overall well-being.

Mental and emotional resilience: Readers are guided in navigating the emotional challenges of menopause, helping them build emotional resilience and maintain robust mental health.

Hormone therapy insights: The book explores the pros and cons of hormone replacement therapy (HRT) and other medical options, allowing readers to make informed decisions about their health.

Sexual health: Changes in sexual desire and intimacy are addressed, with guidance on how to maintain a satisfying and fulfilling sex life during and after menopause.

Life beyond menopause: The book emphasizes that menopause is not an endpoint but a new beginning, providing insight into refocusing on personal goals, relationships, and self-discovery.

Support and community: Connecting with others going through menopause is a vital source of support and encouragement.

Empowerment: Ultimately, "Navigating Menopause" empowers women to take control of their health, make informed decisions, and live life to the fullest during and after this significant phase.

This book is a source of inspiration, knowledge, and practical guidance, enabling women to face menopause with confidence and embrace a life of full bloom.

Embrace menopause with confidence and vitality: Your Journey to Full Bloom.

Menopause is not an ending but a remarkable new chapter in the book of your life. It is a transition that signifies strength, wisdom, and a future brimming with potential. As you approach this transformative period, remember that you are not alone. Millions of women around the world are embarking on this very same journey, each one capable of embracing menopause with confidence and vitality.

Your strength and wisdom:

Menopause is a testament to your strength. It's the culmination of a lifetime of experiences, challenges, and achievements. Your body is undergoing changes, but these changes don't define you. Instead, they are a reflection of the amazing journey you've been on. Embrace your inner strength, for it will carry you through this transition with grace.

The power of knowledge:

Understanding is the key to confidence. Knowledge about the physical, emotional, and psychological aspects of menopause empowers you to navigate this journey with confidence. When you know what to expect, you can make informed decisions and take control of your well-being. The more you know, the more confident you become.

Wellness and vitality:

Menopause is not a time for stagnation but a time for rejuvenation. Prioritize your wellness – physical and emotional. Discover the power of nutrition, exercise, and self-care to keep your vitality alive. These are the tools that will help you bloom even brighter in this new phase of life.

Mental and emotional resilience:

Your emotional health is just as important as your physical health. Menopause can be a rollercoaster of emotions, but remember that your resilience is your greatest asset. You have faced challenges before, and you have triumphed. Use that inner strength to conquer any emotional hurdles.

Hormone therapy as an option:

If needed, consider hormone therapy as an ally on your journey. It's one of the many tools available to help you manage menopausal symptoms. Consult with a healthcare professional to make an informed choice that suits your needs.

Reignite your passion:

Menopause doesn't dim your desires; it refocuses them. Rediscover your passions, explore new interests, and rekindle the flames of love and intimacy. Your vitality is still very much alive, and your life is ready for exciting new chapters.

Community and support:

You are never alone on this journey. Seek the company of fellow women who understand the challenges and joys of menopause. Share your experiences, provide support, and receive the encouragement you deserve. Together, you can navigate this transition with strength and vitality.

Conclusion:

Approach menopause with confidence and vitality, for it is a time of transformation and renewal. Your strength, knowledge, wellness, resilience, and the support of your community are your greatest allies. Embrace this transition as a chance to bloom and thrive. Your journey is not ending; it's just beginning, and it's a journey full of confidence and vitality.

BONUS

REAL FREQUENTLY ASKED QUESTIONS,
EXPERTLY ANSWERED

Q1. What are the best and affordable supplements to take after a full hysterectomy surgery?

Answer: After a hysterectomy, it is essential to consult with a doctor for personalized recommendations. Commonly recommended supplements include:
• Calcium and Vitamin D: To support bone health.
• Iron: To replenish any blood loss during surgery.
• Multivitamins: To ensure adequate intake of essential nutrients.

Q2. Can fatty liver and high cholesterol cause symptoms like dizziness and difficulty walking, and what should be done?

Answer: Yes, these conditions can contribute to such symptoms. If you are experiencing dizziness, headaches, and difficulty walking, here is what you should do:

• Medical Follow-up: Regular consultations with your doctor are essential to monitor and adjust treatment as needed.
• Lifestyle Changes: Adopt a balanced diet low in saturated fats and sugars, engage in physical activity as appropriate, and avoid alcohol and tobacco.
• Manage Symptoms: Work with your doctor to identify causes and management strategies.

Q3. Is gray hair associated with scalp itching, and what can be done?

Answer: Gray hair itself does not typically cause itching, but the scalp can become dry or irritated with age, potentially due to hormonal changes during menopause. To relieve itching:
• Use moisturizing shampoos and conditioners.
• Avoid harsh hair products.
• Consult a dermatologist for further advice if needed.

Q4. Can dry, itchy inner thighs be related to perimenopause, and how can it be treated?

Answer: Yes, hormonal changes during perimenopause can lead to skin dryness and irritation. Treatments include:
• Moisturizing: Use fragrance-free moisturizers.
• Breathable Clothing: Wear loose-fitting fabrics.
• Mild Products: Choose fragrance-free soaps and detergents.
• Hydration: Drink plenty of water.
• Medical Advice: Seek further evaluation if symptoms persist.

Q5. Is inner ear itching a sign of menopause?

Answer: No, inner ear itching is not typically a symptom of menopause. It may be due to allergies, infections, or excessive earwax. Consult a healthcare professional for diagnosis and treatment.

Q6. What should be done if experiencing body and joint pains that recur every 1-2 weeks?

Answer: Persistent body and joint pains could indicate underlying health issues. It is important to:
• Consult a Doctor: For a thorough examination and tests.
• Lifestyle Adjustments: Regular exercise, a balanced diet, and stress management can help alleviate symptoms.

Q7. Could chest pain radiating to the left hand be related to menopause?

Answer: No, such chest pain is not typically associated with menopause. It may be a sign of a heart-related issue. Immediate medical attention is advised, including possible tests like an electrocardiogram (ECG).

Q8. Can pregnancy occur at age 51+, and what could irregular menstrual symptoms indicate?

Answer: While pregnancy at this age is less likely, it is not impossible. Other potential causes include hormonal changes or side effects from medications. Consult a healthcare provider for an accurate diagnosis.

Q9. What should a woman with abdominal pain and no intimate partner for 1.5 years consider?

Answer: This could be related to various issues, including hormonal changes due to menopause. Consult with a healthcare professional for a thorough evaluation and consider support from a therapist for emotional well-being.

Q10. What could cause menstruation to restart after 1.5 years without a period?

Answer: This can be due to hormonal fluctuations, stress, weight changes, or underlying conditions. Medical evaluation is necessary to determine the cause and provide appropriate treatment.

Q11. How can a 40-year-old woman get her period back to conceive?

Answer: Consult a healthcare provider to assess overall health and hormone levels. Treatments or lifestyle adjustments can be recommended based on the diagnosis.

Q12.Is menopause over at age 57 after stopping menstruation at 48?

Answer: Menopause is considered complete after 12 months without menstruation. At 57, it is likely over, but consulting a healthcare provider for personalized advice is recommended.

Q13. What can be done to manage menopause-related weight loss?

Answer: Although menopause usually causes weight gain, some women experience weight loss due to:
• Hormonal Changes
• Stress and Emotional Factors
• Diet and Lifestyle Adjustments
• Health Conditions (e.g., hyperthyroidism)

Consult a healthcare provider for guidance.

Q14. What is the average age for menopause, and what factors influence it?

Answer: Menopause typically occurs between 45-55, with an average age of 51. Influences include genetics, lifestyle factors, and certain health conditions.

Q15. How should waking up at night gasping for breath be managed during menopause?

Answer: • Consult a Healthcare Provider: To rule out conditions like sleep apnea or anxiety disorders.
• Lifestyle Changes: Regular exercise, stress management, and sleep hygiene can help.
• Breathing and Relaxation Techniques: Can reduce symptoms.

Q16. Is there a connection between menopause and halitosis?

Answer: Yes, reduced estrogen can lower saliva production, causing dry mouth and bad breath. Manage it with:
• Oral Hygiene: Floss and brush teeth regularly.
• Hydration and Chewing Sugar-Free Gum: To stimulate saliva.
• Diet Adjustments: Avoid foods that linger, like garlic and alcohol.

Q17. What should be done if a 49-year-old experiences heavy sweating and missed periods without pregnancy?

Answer: This could be related to perimenopause. Other causes might include:
• Hormonal changes
• Anxiety or stress
• Thyroid issues
• Medication side effects
• Other medical conditions (e.g., diabetes)

Consult a healthcare provider for a comprehensive evaluation that includes a physical exam, medical history, and blood tests (e.g., hormone and thyroid function). Discuss potential treatment options and lifestyle changes with your doctor.

Q18. Is body itching related to menopause, and what are the common symptoms?

Answer: Yes, body itching can be associated with menopause due to reduced estrogen levels. Symptoms include:
• Itching on the limbs, neck, face, chest, back, or elbows.
• Tingling, prickling, or numbness.
• Vaginal itching.
• Dry, red, or flaky skin.
• General skin sensitivity.

If the itching persists or becomes severe, seek medical attention for proper treatment and management.

Q19. Can menopause lead to hair loss, and what are the contributing factors?

Answer: Yes, menopause can cause hair loss due to:
• Decreasing estrogen levels, which slow hair growth.
• Increased androgens, such as testosterone, contributing to hair thinning.
• Aging and the natural process of menopause.
• Stress during this period.
• Nutritional deficiencies, like low levels of iron, zinc, or biotin.

Common Hair Loss Patterns:
• Thinning or falling hair on the scalp.
• Widening of the center part.
• Hair loss on the crown or top of the head.
• Excessive shedding.

Management Tips:
• Maintain a diet rich in vitamins and minerals.
• Reduce stress through exercise, meditation, or therapy.
• Use gentle hair care products and avoid excessive heat styling.
• Consult a healthcare provider for personalized advice, including potential hormone replacement therapy (HRT) or other treatments.

Q20. What foods can help regain strength, appetite, and memory in older adults?

Answer: A balanced diet with specific nutrient-rich foods is essential for older adults to regain strength and vitality. Recommended foods include:

1. Protein-Rich Foods:
• Lean meats (chicken, turkey).
• Fatty fish (salmon, mackerel) for omega-3 fatty acids.
• Eggs, legumes, and nuts.

2. Whole Grains:
• Oats, quinoa, brown rice, whole wheat bread.

3. Fruits and Vegetables:
• Leafy greens (spinach, kale).
• Berries (blueberries, strawberries).
• Citrus fruits, tomatoes, broccoli.

4. Healthy Fats:
• Olive oil, avocados, nuts.

5. Dairy:
• Greek yogurt, milk (fortified with vitamin D), moderate amounts of cheese.

6. Hydration:
• Plenty of water, herbal teas, and fresh fruit juices.

Memory-Boosting Foods:
• Blueberries (high in antioxidants).
• Turmeric (contains curcumin with anti-inflammatory benefits).
• Broccoli (rich in vitamin K and antioxidants).
• Pumpkin seeds (contain magnesium, iron, zinc, and copper).

Supplements:
• Vitamin B12 for nerve and brain function.
• Omega-3 fatty acids (e.g., fish oil).
• Vitamin D for bone and muscle health.

Additional Tips:
• Regular, balanced meals.
• Light exercise and mental activities to enhance cognitive health.

APPENDIX

*Additional Resources, Pharmaceutical Dosage
Guidelines, and Recommendations*

A. Additional Resources

Books:

"The Wisdom of Menopause" by Dr. Christiane Northrup

"Menopause Confidential" by Dr. Tara Allmen

"The Menopause Book" by Barbara Kantrowitz and Pat Wingert

Websites and online communities:

Menopause Support Nigeria: A public health enlightenment initiative created to educate, enlighten, and support the public on menopause, its symptoms, and its management.

North American Menopause Society (NAMS): A comprehensive resource for menopause information, research, and support.

Women's Health: The U.S. Department of Health and Human Services offers a wealth of information on women's health, including menopause.

Menopause Matters: A UK-based website providing evidence-based information and support for women experiencing menopause.

Support groups:

Check with local healthcare providers, women's clinics, or hospitals for information on menopause support groups in your area.

Mobile Apps:

"My Menopause Journey" (Available on iOS and Android) - A comprehensive app to track menopausal symptoms, manage wellness, and access relevant articles and resources.

B.Pharmaceutical Dosage Guidelines

Hormone replacement therapy (HRT) dosage guidelines:

It is essential to consult with a healthcare professional before starting HRT. Dosages will vary based on individual needs, medical history, and the type of HRT being prescribed. The following are general guidelines and should not replace personalized medical advice:

- **Estrogen therapy:** Common starting doses for oral estrogen range from 0.5 to 2 mg/day. Transdermal patches or creams may be prescribed at varying doses. Follow your healthcare provider's guidance closely.
- **Progestin therapy:** The choice of progestin type and dosage varies, depending on the individual's health, and on whether the individual still has a uterus. A typical dose of medroxyprogesterone acetate is 2.5 to 10 mg/day for 10 to 14 days of the cycle.
- **Bioidentical hormone therapy:** Dosages can vary widely depending on the formulation and individual needs. Compounded bioidentical hormones should be prescribed and monitored by a healthcare professional.

C.Recommendations

Regular check-ups: Schedule regular check-ups with your healthcare provider to monitor your menopausal progress and discuss any concerns or adjustments to your treatment plan.

Lifestyle modifications: Continue to prioritize a healthy lifestyle, including a balanced diet, regular exercise, stress management, and adequate sleep.

Ongoing learning: Stay informed about the latest research and developments in menopause management to make informed decisions about your health.

Supportive networks: Engage with local or online support groups and communities to share your experiences, seek advice, and offer support to others.

Holistic approaches: Explore complementary therapies such as acupuncture, yoga, and meditation in consultation with your healthcare provider.

Remember that this appendix is meant to provide additional resources, general pharmaceutical dosage guidelines, and recommendations. Still, individual medical advice should always be sought from a healthcare professional who understands your unique needs and medical history.

For the most current information on pharmaceutical dosages and treatments, consult your healthcare provider or a menopause specialist.

BIBLIOGRAPHY

1. General Information on Menopause:

The North American Menopause Society (NAMS). (2014). The 2012 hormone therapy position statement of The North American Menopause Society. *Menopause, 21*(9), [887-902].

2. Hormone Replacement Therapy (HRT):

Manson, J. E., & Bassuk, S. S. (2018). The menopausal transition and postmenopausal hormone therapy. *In UpToDate. Waltham, MA: UpToDate Inc.*

Stuenkel, C. A., & Pinkerton, J. V. (2018). Management of common menopausal symptoms. *In UpToDate. Waltham, MA: UpToDate Inc.*

Haufe, A, et al. J Endocr. Soc.2023.PMID:37091307

3. Lifestyle and Wellness During Menopause:

Thurston, R. C., & Santoro, N. (2017). Mind the gap: What do we know about risk and protective factors for cognitive decline during the menopausal transition? *Menopause, 24*(8), [833-834].

Avis, N. E., & Crawford, S. L. (2018). Will the new decade bring clarity about menopausal hormone therapy and cognitive outcomes? *Menopause, 25*(1), [3-4].

4. Emotional and Psychological Resilience:

Woods, N. F., Cray, L., Mitchell, E. S., & Hohensee, C. (2018). The Menopause Experience: A Contemporary Analysis. *Journal of Women's Health, 27*(5), [493-501].

Bromberger, J. T., Schott, L. L., Avis, N. E., & Crawford, S. L. (2015). The Menopause Transition and Sexual Function: The Study of Women's Health Across the Nation (SWAN). *Journal of Women's Health, 24*(5), [361-368].

5. Sexual Health During Menopause:

Shifren, J. L. (2016). Sexual problems in women: Menopause and beyond. *In UpToDate. Waltham, MA: UpToDate Inc.*

Nappi, R. E., & Cucinella, L. (2014). Advances in pharmacotherapy for the treatment of female sexual dysfunction. *Expert Opinion on Pharmacotherapy, 15*(9), [1227-1236].

6. Holistic Approaches and Complementary Therapies:

Elkins, G., Marcus, J., Stearns, V., Perfect, M. M., & Rajab, M. H. (2007). Efficacy and safety of mindfulness-based stress reduction for vasomotor symptoms in breast cancer survivors: a randomized, controlled trial. Menopause, 14(6), 995-1009.

Borrelli, F., Ernst, E. (2010). Alternative and complementary therapies for the menopause. *Maturitas, 66*(4), [333-343].

7. Support and Community for Women:

Avis, N. E., Colvin, A., & Bromberger, J. T. (2008). Change in health-related quality of life over the menopausal transition in a multiethnic cohort of middle-aged women: Study of Women's Health Across the Nation (SWAN). *Menopause, 15*(5), [832-838].

Gold, E. B., & Sternfeld, B. (2002). Relation of demographic and lifestyle factors to symptoms in a multi-racial/ethnic population of women 40–55 years of age. *American Journal of Epidemiology, 156*(6), [522-531].